Hypertension in ...g..a..y

Hypertension in Pregnancy

DAVID CHURCHILL
Consultant Obstetrician and Gynaecologist
Good Hope Hospital, Sutton Coldfield

and

D GARETH BEEVERS
Professor of Medicine
University of Birmingham

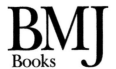

© BMJ Books 1999
BMJ Books is an imprint of the BMJ Publishing Group

First published in 1999
by BMJ Books, BMA House, Tavistock Square,
London WC1H 9JR

British Library Cataloguing in Publication Data

A catalogue record for this book is available from the British Library

ISBN 0-7279-0920-7

Typeset by Apek Typesetters, Nailsea, Bristol
Printed and bound by Latimer Trend, Plymouth

Contents

Contributors

Karen Brackley   Sub-specialist Registrar in Fetal Medicine, Birmingham Women's Hospital.

Mark D Kilby   Senior Lecturer/Honorary Consultant in Fetal Medicine, University of Birmingham.

David I Thomas   Consultant Anaesthetist, Good Hope Hospital, Sutton Coldfield.

Preface

In the eighteenth and nineteenth centuries women who had completed a successful pregnancy went through a process of churching in which they were welcomed back into the community and gave thanks for their survival. The christening of the baby came later. In those days the maternal mortality rates were high and women knew it. Similarly, the perinatal and infant mortality rates were horrifying, even in the most affluent of families. The high fertility rates in those days were in part related to the knowledge that many pregnancies would lead to stillbirth, early neonatal death or sickly children; a tendency still seen today in some developing countries. The American physician and essayist Oliver Wendell Holmes and the Hungarian obstetrician Ignac Semmelweis had both observed that many of the maternal deaths were due to infection. Both made the then startling suggestion that obstetricians and midwives should remove their dirty and often bloodstained outer clothing and wash their hands before delivering a baby. Thus infection as a cause of maternal and infant death gradually declined, aided later by the arrival of the antibiotic era. The history of obstetrics over the past 50 years has been characterised by a steady decline in maternal and perinatal mortality due to infection, thromboembolic events and intrapartum mechanical problems. During this time, the hypertensive disorders have thus become relatively more important and now represent a major challenge for both obstetricians and midwives.

The idea for this book was conceived whilst embarking upon a major study of blood pressure measurement in pregnancy. Whilst carrying out our jointly run clinic for pregnant women suffering from hypertension, we had many debates regarding the diagnosis, investigation and treatment of individual patients. It became clear that despite avidly reading much of the published work across the world, decisions on the clinical management of these patients remained far from straightforward.

There are many texts dealing with hypertension in pregnancy and many more chapters on the subject in standard obstetric and medical books. The emphasis within these books and chapters is rightly focused on the pre-eclampsia syndrome. We do not wish to detract from any of these publications and have ourselves found them valuable sources of information. However, many of the large publications are written from the point of view of the clinical scientist, who is usually involved in researching a particular aspect of pre-eclampsia. Information relevant to clinical practice has to be distilled from the scientific data and theories.

The aim of this book is to provide obstetricians, midwives, and general practitioners with a more didactic approach to the clinical management of patients with hypertension at whatever stage this may develop during their pregnancy. We have tried to base our ideas upon sound evidence, as presented in the scientific literature, and have tried not to distort this evidence but to produce a balanced account of the "state of the art". Undoubtedly, when trying to review and précis a vast body of data one has to make certain value judgements, but we hope that we have not over-simplified the issues. We have included what we feel are the main areas of interest today and possibly for the future.

We do not claim to provide all the answers regarding the hypertensive disorders of pregnancy but hope to produce a guide or framework for managing these particular patients. Whether this aim is achieved, we leave to the judgement of our readers. Like the other texts on hypertension in pregnancy, this book will inevitably in large part concentrate upon pre-eclampsia, for this is the condition causing most morbidity and mortality. But we hope not to neglect the other hypertensive conditions, which do occur with varying degrees of frequency in pregnancy. While they may not hold such poor prognoses as pre-eclampsia, they still cause clinical problems such as intrauterine growth retardation and difficulties in diagnosing superimposed pre-eclampsia.

It is widely believed that pre-eclampsia is one of a group of disorders which are characterised by placental ischaemia, possibly resulting from a primary defect in vascular endothelium of the placenta. The pathophysiology of the condition is still not fully understood and the discovery of its aetiology is some way off. It is therefore necessary to rely upon clinical symptoms and signs to assign the particular diagnosis to an individual woman. The many variants of the condition mean that the clinicians looking after pregnant women have to be vigilant and aware at all times.

It has almost become ritualistic when writing or talking about hypertension in pregnancy to quote the latest figures from the last triennial report into maternal mortality. We will refrain from doing this but merely present a table at the beginning of the book. This, we feel, speaks for itself. Readers who wish to delve further into maternal mortality are referred to the reports themselves.

We will refer those readers interested in taking the study of this group of disorders to greater depths to other texts.

All that remains to be said is that the hypertensive disorders of pregnancy are truly fascinating in a scientific and clinical sense. They present a particular challenge to all practising in the field of obstetrics and midwifery. We hope that readers find this book both enjoyable and informative, and gain something from it which may help them when managing women with pregnancies complicated by hypertension.

DC
DGB

Causes of direct maternal deaths, percentage of direct deaths and rates per 1 000 000 maternities: United Kingdom, 1985–93. Reproduced with permission from Hibbard BM. Report on confidential enquiries into maternal deaths in the United Kingdom 1991–1993, HMSO: London, 1996.

Triennia		Thrombosis and thrombo-embolism[a]	Hypertensive disorders of pregnancy	Anaesthesia	Amniotic fluid embolism	Early pregnancy deaths including abortion[b]	Antepartum and postpartum haemorrhage	Genital tract sepsis (excluding abortion)	Genital tract trauma	Other direct deaths	All direct deaths
1985–87	No.	32(3)	27	6	9	22(16)	10	6	6	21	139
	%	23.0	19.4	4.3	6.5	15.8	7.2	4.3	4.3	15.1	100
	Rate	12.8[c]	11.9	2.6	4.0	2.6[d] 7.1[e]	4.4	2.6	2.6	9.2	61.2
1988–90	No.	33(9)	27	4	11	24(15)	22	7	3	14	145
	%	22.8	18.6	2.8	7.6	16.6	15.2	4.8	2.1	9.7	100
	Rate	10.2[c]	11.4	1.7	4.7	3.8[d] 6.4[e]	9.3	3.0	1.3	5.9	61.4
1991–93	No.	35(5)[a]	20	8	10	18(8)	15	9	4	10	129
	%	27.1	15.5	6.2	7.8	14.0	11.6	7.0	3.1	7.8	100
	Rate	13.0[c]	8.6	3.5	4.3	3.5[d] 3.5[e]	6.5	3.9	1.7	4.3	55.7

Note: Rates are calculated per million maternities.
[a] Numbers due to thromboembolism other than pulmonary are given in parentheses.
[b] Numbers due to ectopic pregnancies given in parentheses.
[c] Rate for pulmonary embolism only.
[d] Rate for abortion.
[e] Rate for ectopic pregnancies.

KIV (muffling) versus KV (disappearance of sounds) for the measurement of diastolic pressure in pregnancy: which is the best?

The argument over whether to use muffling or the disappearance of sounds as the level at which diastolic pressure should be read in pregnancy has been raging for some years. The advocates for Korotkov sound IV (KIV) as the level of diastolic pressure in pregnancy argued that the difference between KIV and KV was so great as to make the disappearance of sounds too low to be the true measure of diastolic pressure. In addition they also argued that the disappearance of sounds was often heard down to zero in pregnancy.[8] This has remained the situation for many years. However, a survey of midwives and obstetricians in the UK revealed a more chaotic picture.[9] There was no agreement upon which level, KIV or KV, to use for diastolic pressure and this prompted further investigations to be carried out. A prospective case control study examining the difference between the two sounds in pregnant and age-matched non-pregnant women, found that the gap between KIV and KV in pregnancy was indeed larger, but that the difference itself was only 2 mmHg. The authors concluded that this was unlikely to be clinically significant.[10] Intra-arterial blood pressure measurement studies showed that KV, even in pregnancy, corresponded better to the level of diastolic pressure than did KIV.[11]

Moreover, the disappearance of sounds has several other advantages over muffling. The main one being that there is a reduction in the inter- and intra-observer errors experienced when measuring diastolic pressure to KV as opposed to KIV. It would appear that the arguments surrounding KIV and KV have now been resolved. Recent papers and editorials have firmly stated that KV should be used for the measurement of diastolic pressure in both the pregnant and non-pregnant states.[12-14] This change will bring the UK into line with the USA where the ACOG recommends the use of KV for the measurement of diastolic pressure. This new consistency should help to clear up the confusion and hopefully improve accuracy when taking blood pressure measurements. Where sounds are genuinely heard down to zero then KIV, the onset of muffling, should be used as the measure of diastolic pressure. This fact should be clearly noted in the patient's records to avoid any confusion between observers. However, clinicians measuring blood pressure must be wary. Too great a pressure upon the brachial artery from the stethoscope will cause sounds to be audible down to zero. Therefore good measurement technique must always be paramount, with the observer conscious of the potential mistakes and pitfalls that can occur when measuring an individual's blood pressure.

Practice Point – Measurement of Diastolic Pressure

- Read diastolic pressure at KV
- KV is closer to arterial pressure than KIV
- Reduces intra- and inter-observer variation
- Greater precision
- The difference between KV and KIV is clinically insignificant
- If sounds are heard to zero, then read at KIV but state so in the notes

---

Measuring devices

The mercury sphygmomanometer has been the principal device of blood pressure measurement for many years and is found in almost all antenatal clinics throughout the country. This situation looks set to change and it is possible that within the next few years the European Union may ban the use of mercury in medical equipment. This will force hospitals into using electronic instrumentation in order to take an individual's blood pressure. Obviously observer errors will be removed from the measurement but new problems will be created. Therefore an awareness of the different kinds of measuring devices in use, including the ordinary sphygmomanometer, is important.

The mercury sphygmomanometer

Even though the concept and design of the mercury column is simple, it is important to ensure that the sphygmomanometer is well maintained. The mercury column must be clean and the mercury in continuity along the whole length of the tube when the blood pressure cuff is inflated (i.e. no bubbles). The glass must be clean enough to read the mercury level to the nearest 2 mm mark. Oxidised mercury will often obscure the markings on older machines.

Damaged or wall mounted sphygmomanometers should be replaced with a stand-alone mercury manometer as shown in

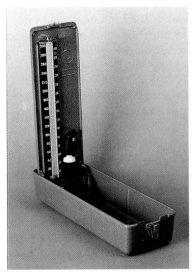

Figure 1.3   The standard mercury manometer is the mainstay machine of blood pressure measurement in the UK. Despite its simplicity it still requires careful maintenance.

Figure 1.3. These manometers are cheap to maintain and if damaged in any permanent way, relatively inexpensive to replace.

The aneroid sphygmomanometer

These devices are popular with GPs, community midwives and district nurses because of their portability. Pressure from the occluding arm cuff is applied to a bellows assembly, which is stretched. The movement in the bellows is transmitted and amplified by a gearing system to drive a pointer. Unfortunately, like all mechanical devices it is subject to errors and they have been found to deviate significantly from the mercury column sphygmomanometer.[15] Ideally these machines should be checked every 6 months and should be returned to the manufacturer for any necessary maintenance. Abnormal blood pressure readings taken with these devices should still be taken seriously although they should be checked against readings made with a mercury sphygmomanometer.

The random zero sphygmomanometer

Because of the problems of observer bias and terminal digit preference, the random zero sphygmomanometer was developed

11

for use in the research setting in order to minimise these two undesirable influences. While the machine does not truly conceal the final resting level of the mercury within the column, it is its unpredictability that enables the observer to take a less biased blood pressure measurement. There have been suggestions that the machine itself contains a systematic error. However, recently an exhaustive investigation of the Hawksley found the machine to have a good degree of accuracy and reliability.[16] Therefore for the purposes of medical research, when as many biases and errors need to be eliminated, the random zero sphygmomanometer (Figure 1.4) is still an acceptable method of measuring blood pressure in the absence of validated automated equipment, and its use should be encouraged in these situations.

Automated blood pressure measuring devices

These machines are relatively expensive and need a lot more maintenance in order to maintain their accuracy. It is also important to understand that many of these devices do not measure blood pressure in the same way as a manual reading with

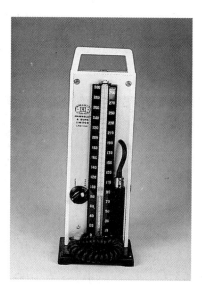

Figure 1.4 The Hawksley random zero sphygmomanometer. The final resting level of mercury in the column is unpredictable. The systolic and diastolic pressures are calculated by subtracting the resting level from the measured levels. In this way biases associated with the observer are reduced.

a mercury manometer, that is to say that sound is not the trigger for measurement. The oscillometric machines, like the Dinamap, sense the onset of pulsation within the brachial artery as the point of systolic pressure and measure the amplitude and frequency of the wave form within the artery as the cuff deflates in order to calculate the mean arterial pressure. From this the device derives the diastolic pressure using an algorithm. Different manufacturers have different algorithms from which they calculate the final blood pressure reading. It is extremely important that before these machines are introduced into clinical practice, they are properly validated on all subsets of patients, including pregnant women.[17] The Spacelabs 90207 is an example of a monitor validated in pregnancy across all ranges of blood pressure (Figure 1.5). However, the calibration of any device needs checking at regular intervals against a set standard, usually the mercury column.

The Omron HEM 705 CP is a validated desktop semi-automatic manometer. This too is an oscillometric machine, which has passed BHS criteria for accuracy and reliability.

Another problem with these types of machines is that at the extremes of the blood pressure range they can become inaccurate. In severe pre-eclampsia it has been shown that some devices may seriously underestimate the basal level of pressure within the circulation.[18] Therefore when managing critically ill patients on the labour ward, the midwives and obstetricians should occasionally

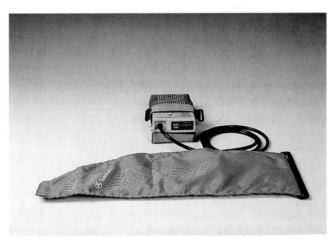

Figure 1.5   The Spacelabs 90207 ambulatory blood pressure measuring has been successfully validated in pregnancy.

check a reading manually, to ensure that the electronic machinery is giving a true reflection of the individual patient's blood pressure. Failure to recognise this underestimation could lead to serious life threatening complications for the patient.

Practice Point – Equipment

- Automated blood pressure devices should be properly validated in all patients, including sub-groups such as pregnant women, and the validation procedure should encompass all levels of blood pressure

---

White coat hypertension

The phenomenon of "white coat hypertension" has been recognised for many years. This can best be described as a rise in a patient's blood pressure when the individual is subjected to a medical environment.[19] The white coat obviously refers to the doctor taking the blood pressure but a similar although somewhat attenuated effect is observed with nurses and midwives. The blood pressure which is recorded, therefore, does not reflect the true level of blood pressure experienced in the patient's normal environment and so may not be a true reflection of an individual's potential pathological state in future years. However, the true significance of white coat hypertension has yet to be determined.[20] There are those who believe that it is an entirely benign condition. Recent evidence shows that it may in fact indicate an individual's susceptibility to cardiovascular morbidity in later life. The time scale of a pregnancy is very much shorter. White coat hypertension in this situation may indeed be benign and unwittingly treating these patients may be unnecessary or even detrimental to their pregnancy. Recognising the phenomenon will ensure that women are not admitted to hospital and treated without good cause.

Ambulatory blood pressure measurement

Home measurement of blood pressure was first tried in the 1970s and it did identify groups of women who were suffering from white coat hypertension. More recently home measurement has been superseded by ambulatory blood pressure monitoring (ABPM). With ABPM, an individual subject wears a small measuring device on a waistband or shoulder strap, which is attached to a cuff situated on the non-dominant arm.[21] The machine is programmed to measure an individual's blood pressure throughout the day, and if required night, usually at 20 or 30 minute intervals. These machines allow individuals to carry on with their normal daily activities and so the measurements recorded will truly reflect the individual's blood pressure. In the general population, as well as detecting white coat hypertension, ambulatory blood pressure monitoring has been shown to be a better predictor of cardiovascular morbidity and mortality when compared to office blood pressure readings.[22, 23] This technique has recently been applied in pregnancy and normal reference ranges for ambulatory blood pressure throughout pregnancy have been calculated.[24, 25] The normal physiological pattern of ambulatory blood pressure throughout a pregnancy seems to be different from that previously described for office blood pressure measurements. Ambulatory blood pressure appears to show a continued rise in both systolic and diastolic pressure levels throughout pregnancy, so that at the end of pregnancy the level of blood pressure is higher than that found in the postnatal period. This is a completely different pattern from that described when office or clinical laboratory measurements are made throughout pregnancy.

The hope that ABPM will provide a better predictor of obstetric outcome remains undecided. Some evidence has been produced to show that there is an inverse relationship between ambulatory blood pressure and birth weight in the normal pregnant population.[26] Work has also been carried out showing that ABPM is possibly a better way of monitoring blood pressure on an outpatient basis, even when compared to measurements made in an antenatal day assessment unit.[27] However, we remain guarded over its usefulness in pregnancy until further reports have been published.

The Measurement and Definition of Proteinuria in Pregnancy

> - "Significant proteinuria is defined as either: (a) one 24 hour collection with a total protein excretion of 300 mg or more per 24 hours or (b) two random clean catch or catheter specimens of urine collected 4 hours or more apart with (i) 2+ (1 g albumin/1) or more on reagent strip, (ii) 1+ (0.3 g albumin/1) if the specific gravity is less than 1030" (ISSHP, 1986)[2]

Screening for proteinuria in the antenatal clinic is universally carried out with dipstix. This method of assessing the level of proteinuria depends upon the observer matching the colour of the test square on a plastic strip to that on a standard chart. Therefore, it can only be at best an estimate of the quantity of protein a woman is losing through her kidneys. The definition for a significant level of proteinuria in pregnancy has been laid down by the ISSHP in its criteria for the diagnosis of pre-eclampsia. The definition of proteinuria states that there must be 2 pluses or more on a dipstix or 1+ when the specific gravity is less than 1030. The significant amounts of proteinuria must be found in two random clean catch specimens of urine or one catheter specimen.

The dipstix themselves have been subjected to tests of reliability and directly compared with quantitative 24 hour urine samples in both normal and hypertensive pregnancies.[28] In the hypertensive pregnancies substantial numbers of false positives and negatives were found; and in addition the inter-observer variations were large. In hypertensive pregnancies they are not to be relied upon as an accurate quantitative measure of protein loss, and when dipstix analysis is positive in a hypertensive's sample, a 24 hour urine collection for total protein measurement should be ordered. These can easily be completed as outpatient tests and do not require a mandatory admission to hospital. Despite these drawbacks, dipstix are a cheap and useful antenatal screen for proteinuria which could be due to either asymptomatic bacteruria or PET. The former is also a cause of preterm labour and worth treating when discovered.

Pregnant women usually bring a urine specimen collected at home to the antenatal clinic. Therefore when proteinuria is identified it is important to enquire how the specimen was taken. If there appears to be a significant amount of proteinuria then a midstream specimen of urine should be taken in the clinic and the test repeated to verify the finding. The specimen should then be sent for microbiological assessment to exclude any infective cause.

The other component of the definition requires the quantification of the amount of proteinuria. If the amount is greater than 300 mg of protein in a 24 hour urine collection, then this is considered abnormal. Obviously the presence of significant levels of proteinuria, in association with hypertension, means that the diagnosis of pre-eclampsia can be made with relative ease. However, proteinuria alone is not necessarily a benign finding. Sometimes significant amounts of proteinuria can precede a rise in blood pressure and the patient may still be at risk of developing pre-eclampsia, even though the blood pressure appears normal. When the diagnosis of pre-eclampsia is made, we try where possible to obtain a 24 hour urine collection in all cases. Quantitative assessment of the level of protein loss can be a useful factor when trying to assess the severity of the disease.

Practice Point – Measurement of Proteinuria

- When abnormal levels of proteinuria are found in the antenatal clinic with samples taken at home, it is important to check this on a clean catch mid-stream specimen. In hypertensives a 24 hour urine save should be ordered to measure the total protein excretion

---

The Classification of the Hypertensive Disorders in Pregnancy

A good classification system should accurately stratify risk and aid the clinician in making rational choices for his or her patients. There have been three principal attempts made at producing a comprehensive and clinically useful classification system for the hypertensive disorders in pregnancy. The system set out by the ISSHP, along with its definitions for hypertension and proteinuria, is the oldest, and has so far withstood the test of time. It is by far the most meaningful breakdown of the various hypertensive disorders in strictly pathological terms. However, it does have its problems, in so far as it does not reflect the true multisystem nature of pre-eclampsia. It is also a cumbersome tool to use in clinical practice. A simpler system has been produced by the National Institutes of Health Working Party in America (NIHWP).[5] This is much more user friendly but also fails to reflect the true multisystem nature of PET. The third and final major classification system is that produced by the Australasian Society for the Study of Hypertension in Pregnancy (ASSHP).[29] The definition of PET is based purely on blood pressure and if the criteria are met after 20 weeks' gestation all patients are categorised as suffering from PET albeit of different degrees with regards to severity. All of the systems will be briefly reviewed in order to present the reader with a comprehensive and hopefully understandable appreciation of the various merits and pitfalls of each system.

ISSHP classification of the hypertensive disorders in pregnancy[2]

The system as defined by the International Society is shown below:

- (A) Gestational hypertension and/or proteinuria
    1 Gestational hypertension (without proteinuria)
    2 Gestational proteinuria (without hypertension)
    3 Gestational proteinuric hypertension (pre-eclampsia)
- (B) Chronic hypertension and chronic renal disease (women found to have hypertension or proteinuria at the first visit before 20 weeks' gestation in the absence of trophoblastic disease, presumed to have either chronic hypertension or chronic renal disease)
    1 Chronic hypertension (without proteinuria)
    2 Chronic renal disease (proteinuria and hypertension)
    3 Chronic hypertension with superimposed pre-eclampsia
- (C) Unclassified hypertension and/or proteinuria (hypertension at first booking > 20 weeks, during labour or the puerperium, where information is insufficient to permit classification)
    1 Unclassified hypertension (without proteinuria)
    2 Unclassified proteinuria (without hypertension)
    3 Unclassified proteinuric hypertension (pre-eclampsia)
This classification can be altered if after pregnancy the hypertension/proteinuria persists to either chronic hypertension or renal disease, or superimposed pre-eclampsia
- (D) Eclampsia

The system is widely used by those carrying out research into hypertension in pregnancy. Because of its precision it makes communication between research workers more meaningful. Publications on the hypertensive disorders of pregnancy should be explicit in which definitions and classification system they use in order to categorise their subjects. This is often not the case. If authors fail to make clear exactly which condition it is they are investigating then the results, which may seem highly significant on paper are much less significant when applied to everyday clinical life.

NIH Working Party classification of the hypertensive disorders in pregnancy[5]

- (A) Chronic hypertension
- (B) Pre-eclampsia–eclampsia
- (C) Pre-eclampsia superimposed on chronic hypertension
- (D) Transient hypertension

The NIHWP classification system is simpler than that produced on behalf of the ISSHP. Its major advantage is that the prognosis for each patient category is broadly understood by clinicians all over the world. Transient hypertension equates with gestational hypertension without proteinuria, according to the ISSHP criteria and is understood to be a mainly benign condition. The simplicity of the system means some loss of precision considering the varied presentations of pre-eclampsia.

It is reasonably argued, however, that neither the ISSHP nor the NIHWP classifications reflect the truly multisystem nature and presentation of the disease pre-eclampsia. Their reliance upon proteinuria being included in the definition of PET leads to the exclusion of women who have other characteristics of PET, i.e. thrombocytopenia, abnormal liver function tests, growth restriction of the fetus, and who would, by common clinical consent, be said to be suffering from pre-eclampsia. The ASSHP system attempted to rectify this problem.

The ASSHP classification system of hypertension in pregnancy[29]

Pre-eclampsia is defined as the development of hypertension after 20 weeks' gestation, in individuals with no known history of hypertension or renal disease. It removes the requirement for the presence of proteinuria in order to make the diagnosis. Pre-eclampsia thus defined is then sub-classified as laid out below:

- Mild
  —Hypertension with or without hyperuricaemia
- Severe
  —Systolic blood pressure >170 mmHg or diastolic BP >110 mmHg, or
  —Maternal organ dysfunction, such as:
  —Haematological, haemolysis or thrombocytopenia $<150 \times 10^6/l$, or
—Proteinuria, >300 mg per day or $>2+$ on dipstix testing, or

19

—Renal impairment, raised serum creatinine, or

—Liver abnormalities with or without severe epigastric or right upper quadrant pain, or

—Neurological, visual scotomata, severe headaches accompanied by hyperreflexia, hyperreflexia with sustained clonus

• Super-imposed PET

  —The development of proteinuria or hyperuricaemia on top of essential hypertension during the second half of pregnancy

This system reflects fully the multisystem nature of the disease pre-eclampsia and the stratification of risk associated with all its presentations. However, by discarding the need for proteinuria as a component of the diagnosis, it leaves out probably the best marker of disease severity, and therefore of perinatal mortality. This in turn could lead to confusion over the term mild pre-eclampsia which equates to gestational hypertension in ISSHP and transient hypertension in the NIH system resulting in the over-treatment of some women.

Suggested alternative systems

The problem with all these definition and classification systems lies with the group of women classified as having gestational/transient hypertension (mild hypertension ASSHP). Within this group there are women with latent essential hypertension, physiological hypertension and non-proteinuric hypertension, all with different prognoses.

Therefore there have been suggestions that these systems should be abandoned and the definition and classification of women with hypertension in pregnancy should be solely based upon the level of maternal blood pressure. Redman and Jefferies[30] used their Oxford dataset to devise a definition for pre-eclampsia based purely on blood pressure changes and obstetric outcome. After settling on their definition, they then tested it upon a different set of women and found a good correlation with obstetric outcome. Their definition is based upon a combination of absolute levels of blood pressure and incremental rises from a baseline in the first half of pregnancy. The definition states that, the combination of: (1) a first antenatal visit diastolic blood pressure less than 90 mmHg, (2) a subsequent increase of at least 25 mmHg during pregnancy and (3) to a maximum reading of >90 mmHg diastolic blood pressure; should lead to the diagnosis of pre-eclampsia, whether or not it is associated with proteinuria.

The definition was tested on a different multi-ethnic population in Birmingham and was found to select out with more precision women with proteinuric pre-eclampsia and having a poorer obstetric outcome.[31]

The simplicity of the Redman and Jefferies definition has an inherent attraction, but it is not yet in widespread use.

The most recent attempt to clarify the situation has come from researchers in Australia.[32] They examined all three main classification systems, applying them to a cohort of over 1000 consecutive women who had hypertension in pregnancy and had been referred to a joint specialist clinic. By the ASSHP criteria, 77% of women were diagnosed with PET, of which 19% had severe PET. Both the NIH and ISSHP systems classified 16% of women as having pre-eclampsia and 71% as having transient or gestational hypertension. The NIH and ISSHP systems defined a much higher risk group for both maternal and fetal outcome overall when compared to the ASSHP criteria without its stratification. However, when compared to severe PET–ASSHP, there was generally good agreement between all three systems regarding maternal and fetal risk. Arising from this paper, Brown proposed a new classification system, combining the best features of all three, and reflecting the multisystem nature of the disease process, the differing stratification of risk and removing any confusion over terminology. It seems to us to be an inherently sensible and clinically practical solution to a problematic area. It is set out below, as described by Brown:

- Pre-eclampsia

  De novo hypertension arising after 20 weeks' gestation returning to normal within 3 months postpartum and one or more of
  —Proteinuria ⩾ 300 mg/day or dipstix result persistently ⩾ 1g/l
  —Renal insufficiency
  —Liver disease: AST 40 IU/l or severe epigastric or right upper quadrant pain or both
  —Neurological problems: convulsions (eclampsia), hyperreflexia with clonus or severe headaches with hyperreflexia
  —Haematological disturbances: thrombocytopenia or haemolysis or both
  —Retardation of fetal growth

- Gestational hypertension

  De novo hypertension after 20 weeks' gestation without any feature of pre-eclampsia, returning to normal within 3 months postpartum

● Chronic hypertension

—Essential hypertension, blood pressure > 140 mmHg systolic or > 90 mmHg diastolic or both before conception or during the first half of pregnancy without an apparent secondary cause or evidence of white coat hypertension
—Secondary hypertension

Summary

It is vitally important that blood pressure measurements are made with a high degree of accuracy. The technique of measurement as set out by the BHS and NHA should be followed meticulously. All operators in the field of obstetrics should recognise the damage that can be done by misdiagnosing a woman either as hypertensive or alternatively as normotensive because of sloppy blood pressure measurement technique.

To date the three most important classification systems in use are those laid down first by the ISSHP, secondly by the NIH working party and thirdly by the ASSHP. The latter two are more clinically applicable and user friendly. However, clinicians and researchers should be explicit in the terminology they use and in that situation the ISSHP classification may be more suitable.

Practice Point – Clinical Practice

● Be wary of the many varied presentations of pre-eclampsia. At first sight the symptoms and signs may not fit the classical definitions or classification systems

---

Classically, pre-eclampsia should refer to the dyad of hypertension and proteinuria after 20 weeks' gestation. However, it should be remembered that the disease process could occur without proteinuria but with other features. Gestational hypertension should refer to raised blood pressure alone in the second half of pregnancy. This diagnosis can only be made retrospectively, as determining which patient will develop proteinuria or other abnormalities is impossible to predict with any degree of certainty. Chronic essential hypertension should be applied to those women who have raised blood pressure prior to 20 weeks' gestation and where another non-pregnant cause cannot be found. As well as the measurement of blood pressure, dipstick testing of the urine should be carried out as accurately as possible and whenever the disease pre-eclampsia is suspected, if the clinical condition allows, a 24 hour urine save should be carried out to quantify the total loss of protein. This along with all the other investigations will then allow an accurate diagnosis and assessment of the severity of the clinical condition to be made in each individual. Only then can an appropriate clinical course of action be planned for each patient.

For the future, this may all change and the system proposed by Brown and Buddle has lots to commend it to both the clinical and scientific community alike. For sure the debate will begin, but we feel that the system proposed may very well provide the best of all worlds given the current state of knowledge. It will more importantly be a great help to clinicians in identifying the "at risk" woman, while at the same time recognising the multisystem nature of the disease pre-eclampsia. We commend this system for use in clinical practice.

The principles of good blood pressure measurement technique are:

- Follow the guidance from the British Hypertension Society
- Use clean, well-maintained machinery
- Relax the patient as much as possible
- Choose the correct cuff size
- Deflate the bladder at 2 mmHg each second and no faster
- Avoid observer errors such as terminal digit preference
- Read the systolic and diastolic pressures to the nearest 2 mm mark
- Use the disappearance of sounds, Korotkov V, to measure off diastolic pressure

---

References

1 McCowan LME, Buist RG, North RA, Gamble G. Perinatal morbidity in chronic hypertension. *Br J Obstet Gynaecol* 1996;**103**:123–9.
2 Davey DA, MacGillivray I. The classification and definition of the hypertensive disorders of pregnancy. *Am J Obstet Gynecol* 1988;**158**:892–8.

3 Friedman EA, Neff RK. Pregnancy outcome as related to hypertension, oedema and proteinuria. In: Lindheimer MD, Katz AI, Zuspan FP, eds. *Hypertension in pregnancy*. New York: John Wiley, 1976.

4 Hughes EC ed., *Obstetric-gynecologic terminology*. Philadelphia: FA Davis, 1972, 422–3

5 National High Blood Pressure Education Program Working Group Report on High Blood Pressure in Pregnancy. *Am J Obstet Gynecol* 1990;**163**:1689–712.

6 Feher M, Harris St John, Lant A. Blood pressure measurement by junior hospital doctors–a gap in medical education. *Health Trends* 1992;**24**:59–61.

7 O'Brien E, Petrie J, Littler W *et al*. The British Hypertension Society Protocol for the evaluation of automated and semi-automated blood pressure measuring devices with special reference to ambulatory systems. *J Hypertens* 1990;**8**:607–19.

8 MacGillivray I, Rose G, Rowe B. Blood pressure survey in pregnancy. *Clin Sci* 1969;**37**:395–407.

9 Perry IJ, Wilkinson LS, Shinton RA, Beevers DG. Conflicting views on the measurement of blood pressure in pregnancy. *Br J Obstet Gynaecol* 1991;**98**:241–3.

10 Perry IJ, Stewart BA, Brockwell J *et al*. Recording diastolic blood pressure in pregnancy. *Br Med J* 1990;**301**:1198.

11 Brown MA, Whitworth JA. Recording diastolic blood pressure in pregnancy. *Br Med J* 1991;**303**:120–1

12 Shennan A, Gupta M, Halligan A, Taylor DJ, de Sweit M. Lack of reproducibility in pregnancy of Korotkoff phase IV as measured by mercury sphygmomanometry. *Lancet* 1996;**347**:139–42.

13 Rubin P. Measuring diastolic blood pressure in pregnancy. *Br Med J* 1996;**313**:4–5.

14 Franx A, van der Post JAM, van Montfrans GA, Bruinse HW, Visser GHA. The fourth sound of Korotkoff in pregnancy: a myth? *Lancet* 1996;**347**:841.

15 O'Brien E, O'Malley K. *Essentials of blood pressure measurement*. Edinburgh: Churchill Livingstone, 1981:19.

16 Brown WCB, Kennedy S, Inglis GC, Murray LS, Lever AF. Mechanisms by which the Hawksley random zero sphygmomanometer underestimates blood pressure and produces a non random distribution of RZ values. *J Hum Hypertens* 1997;**11**:75–94.

17 Shennan A, Halligan A, Gupta M, Taylor D, de Sweit M. Oscillometric blood pressure measurements in severe pre-eclampsia: a validation of the Spacelabs 90207. *Br J Obstet Gynaecol* 1996;**103**:171–2.

18 Quinn M. Automated blood pressure measurement devices: a potential source of morbidity in pre-eclampsia. *Am J Obstet Gynecol* 1994;**170**:1303–7.

19 Mancia G, Bertinieri G, Grassi G *et al*. Alerting reaction and rise in blood pressure during measurement by physician and nurse. *Hypertension* 1987;**9**:209–15.

20 Mancia G, Parati G. Clinical significance of white coat hypertension. *Hypertension* 1990;**16**:624–6.

21 Halligan A, O'Brien E, Walshe J, O'Malley K, Darling M. Clinical application of ambulatory blood pressure measurement in pregnancy. *J Hypertens* 1991;**9** (Suppl 8): S75–7.

22 Perloff D, Sokolow M, Cowan R. The prognostic value of ambulatory blood pressures. *J Am Med Assoc* 1983;**249**:2729–8.

23 Perloff D, Sokolow M, Cowan R, Juster RP. Prognostic value of ambulatory blood pressure measurements: a further analysis. *J Hypertens* 1989;**7** (Suppl 3): S3–10.

24 Halligan A, O'Brien E, O'Malley K *et al*. Twenty four hour ambulatory blood pressure measurement in a primigravid population. *J Hypertens* 1993;**11**:869–73.

25 Churchill D, Beevers DG. Differences between office and ambulatory blood pressure measurement during pregnancy. *Obstet Gynecol* 1996;**88**:455–61.

26 Churchill D, Perry IJ, Beevers DG. Ambulatory blood pressure in pregnancy and fetal growth. *Lancet* 1997;**349**:7–10.

27 Peek M, Shennan A, Halligan A *et al.* Hypertension in pregnancy: which method of blood pressure measurement is most predictive of outcome? *Obstet Gynecol* 1996;**88**:1030–3.

28 Kuo VS, Koumantakis G, Gallery EDM. Proteinuria and its assessment in normal and hypertensive pregnancy. *Am J Obstet Gynecol* 1992;**167**:723–8.

29 Australasian Society for the Study of Hypertension in Pregnancy. Consensus statement–management of hypertension in pregnancy, executive summary. *Med J Aust* 1993; **158**:700–2.

30 Redman CWG, Jefferies M. Revised definition of pre-eclampsia. *Lancet* 1988; **i**:809–12.

31 Perry IJ, Beevers DG. The definition of pre-eclampsia. *Br J Obstet Gynaecol* 1994;**101**:587–91.

32 Brown MA, Buddle ML. What's in a name? Problems with the classification of hypertension in pregnancy. *J Hypertens* 1997;**15**:1049–54.

2 Prevalence of the Hypertensive Disorders of Pregnancy and Their Risk

DG BEEVERS AND D CHURCHILL

What Is Hypertension?

At a pathophysiological level hypertension is simply a raised blood pressure within the arterial tree due to vasoconstriction and narrowing of the small arterioles, leading to an increase in peripheral resistance to blood flow.[1] In the non-pregnant state it is one of three common risk factors for the premature development of heart attack and stroke, the other two being cigarette smoking and hyperlipidaemia. Hypertension is therefore largely a problem of older people affecting between 20 and 40% of the population.[2] It is clear therefore that hypertension in pregnancy and hypertension in men and women aged 50 years or more are qualitatively and quantitatively different. The atherothrombotic complications of hypertension (heart attacks and strokes) are very rare in pregnancy or indeed in pre-menopausal women. The tendency for clinicians to extrapolate their understanding of hypertension from non-pregnancy states to pregnancy has been the source of much confusion.

The classification of hypertension adopted by the World Health Organisation and other bodies was introduced for use in the non-pregnant state; it is however generally accepted and can therefore be used for pregnancy as well.

Classification of Hypertension Used in Non-pregnant Patients

- Diastolic blood pressure 90 mmHg or more — Diastolic hypertension
- Systolic blood pressure 160 mmHg or more with diastolic pressure below 90 mmHg — Isolated systolic hypertension
- Systolic blood pressure between 140 and 159 mmHg with diastolic pressure below 90 mmHg — Borderline isolated systolic hypertension
- Blood pressure below 140/90 mmHg — Normotension

Of those individuals classified as having hypertension, the majority (around 97%) are classified as having essential hypertension with no underlying renal or adrenal cause.[3] Essential hypertension is thought to be related to the interplay of genetic factors and lifestyle influences, including salt intake, obesity and other factors.[2] In the remaining 3% of patients, underlying medical conditions can be identified including glomerulonephritis, pyelonephritis, renal artery stenosis, phaeochromocytoma and primary hyperaldosteronism. These patients are classified as having secondary hypertension.

Practice Point – Incidence

- 97% of individuals with chronic hypertension have essential hypertension

Raised Blood Pressure in Pregnancy

In pregnant women the importance of different levels of blood pressure is significantly different from that in the non-pregnant state although the dividing line of 140/90 mmHg is still employed. However, mildly raised blood pressures in pregnancy, which are persistently between 140 and 150 mmHg (systolic), and 90 and 100 mmHg (diastolic), uncomplicated by proteinuria, do not appear to carry an adverse prognosis for the baby or for the mother, at least in the short term.

As stated in Chapter 1, there are a great many variations in the classification of the various hypertensive disorders of pregnancy. In particular the significance of "transient" or "gestational" or "pregnancy induced" hypertension is uncertain. There is an increasing view that this condition may be a very mild version of pre-eclampsia, which is not associated with proteinuria, and where the obstetrical outlook is not significantly different from normal. Prevalence figures of the various hypertensive syndromes of pregnancy are hard to come by, partly because of variations in diagnostic criteria, unsystematic obstetrical record keeping and the increasing survival rates following early delivery in women who in the past may have progressed to develop florid pre-eclampsia or even eclampsia. Similarly the outcome in relation to the various hypertensive disorders of pregnancy is variable, depending on the nature of the population studied, the quality of antenatal and intrapartum care, the availability of expert neonatal care, as well as the accuracy of recording. An example of the confusion in diagnostic criteria is provided by the following hypothetical case. A nulliparous woman presenting for medical care for the first time, at 22 weeks of gestation with a blood pressure of 145/95 mmHg with no proteinuria and with no previous blood pressure readings, will be classified as having gestational or transient hypertension, or possibly mild pre-eclampsia, but only if her blood pressure is recorded to be below 140/90 mmHg 7 weeks following delivery of the baby. The final diagnosis is therefore retrospective.

A recent paper from Australia provides some very useful data on the prevalence of the various hypertensive disorders of pregnancy, in relation to two different criteria for diagnosis.[4] The differences in criteria are mainly related to the different interpretations of gestational or transient hypertension mentioned earlier.

The Australian series reviewed 1183 consecutive women with hypertension in pregnancy who had been referred for joint obstetrician/physician care at St George's Hospital, Sydney. This represents 6.7% of nearly 18 000 pregnancies at their hospital. Assuming this includes all hypertensive pregnancies, one can conclude that the overall prevalence of the various hypertensive disorders of pregnancy is between 6 and 7%. This figure is in keeping with data from other centres when combining data from primiparous and multiparous women. The authors subdivided their patients according to two different criteria. The first were the criteria of the Australasian Society for the Study of Hypertension in Pregnancy (ASSHP) (Table 2.1).[5]

The classification of the hypertensive disorders of pregnancy using the criteria of the USA National High Blood Pressure

Table 2.1   Prevalence of the hypertensive disorders of pregnancy encountered in 18 000 consecutive pregnancies by ASSHP criteria

	No.	%
Mild pre-eclampsia	502	2.8
Severe pre-eclampsia	323	1.8
Pre-eclampsia on essential hypertension	82	0.5
Essential hypertension only	223	1.3
Secondary (mainly renal) hypertension	53	0.3
All	**1183**	**6.7**

Education Working Group (NHBPEP) and the series by Davey and MacGillivray[6] adopted by the International Society for the Study of Hypertension in Pregnancy (ISSHP), can be used to classify the same patients.[7] The main differences are the interpretation of rises in blood pressure not associated with proteinuria (Table 2.2).

The prevalence of the rarer syndromes in pregnancy is difficult to calculate because no single hospital will encounter enough cases, and specialist centres tend to see more patients with rare diseases. For example, in the antenatal hypertension clinic at City Hospital, Birmingham, five of the 450 patients seen since 1980 had aortic coarctation, this reflecting the interest in adult congenital heart disease of one of the consultant cardiologists of that hospital.

Classification

- The main difference between the classification systems lies with the prevalence of "gestational" or "transient" hypertension.

Table 2.2   Prevalence of hypertensive disorders of pregnancy encountered in 18 000 consecutive pregnancies by NHBPEP/ISSHP criteria

	No.	%
Gestational/transient hypertension	718	4.1
Pre-eclampsia	154	0.9
Pre-eclampsia on essential hypertension	35	0.2
Essential hypertension	223	1.3
Secondary (mainly renal) hypertension	53	0.3
All	**1183**	**6.7**

High-risk Groups

Parity

Pre-eclampsia is commoner in first pregnancies. In the British Perinatal Mortality survey the prevalence of moderate and severe pre-eclampsia in primigravidae was 13.5% compared with 7.1% in multiparae.[8] This prevalence falls if there is longer sexual cohabitation with the father.[9] Maternal age is an important factor also and is clearly related to parity. Pre-eclampsia is also very common in very young women, particularly related to concealed pregnancy and poor antenatal care, with an important contribution from low social class.

Pre-eclampsia is, however, commonest in women over the age of 30 years in part because of associated multiparity and differences in social class. As with first pregnancy, the prevalence of pre-eclampsia is lower if there is a longer duration of sexual cohabitation.[9] If second or subsequent pregnancies are by a new sexual partner, the pre-eclampsia rates more closely resemble those of primiparous women, but again with relative protection, if there is a longer period of sexual cohabitation.

Inheritance

There is no doubt that pre-eclampsia runs in families. Part of this familial concordance is likely to be due to lifestyle factors but there is now reliable evidence that genetic factors are also operative. However, this effect may in part be related to the genetic inheritance of primary or essential hypertension. Reliable data on the rates of pre-eclampsia in women, their mothers and their mother-in-law do demonstrate a genuine genetic inheritance, possibly by a single gene on the maternal side. Thus pre-eclampsia is unrelated to the family history of the husband.[10, 11]

Twin pregnancies

Severe pre-eclampsia is five times commoner in twin pregnancies than in singletons, with a prevalence of up to 29%.[12] It is probable that pre-eclampsia is commoner in dizygotic twin pregnancies than in monozygotic twins. These data are however influenced by the trend for twin pregnancies to show a similar familial concordance, which might be seen in singleton pregnancies in the same family.

Racial origin

Whilst essential hypertension is commoner in women of African origin when compared to Europeans there is little convincing evidence that there is any genuine racial difference in pre-eclampsia rates, after allowing for the differences in chronic essential hypertension.[13] Any differences in pre-eclampsia seen in the various racial groups may in fact be explained by differences in maternal height, weight (both underweight and overweight), age and possible differences in social class.

Previous essential hypertension

Reliable data on the effects of prior essential hypertension are difficult to obtain, mainly because young women of childbearing age tend not to have had their blood pressures measured until they become pregnant. However, in the Australian series of 1183 consecutive hypertensive pregnancies, 305 women were classified as having essential hypertension and 92 (27%) of these developed superimposed pre-eclampsia.[4] Using the American criteria in the same series, however, this figure falls to 14%. Both these figures are substantially higher than those for pre-eclampsia in women who were previously normotensive.

Oral contraceptive use

There are no reliable data on whether women who sustain a significant rise in blood pressure whilst taking the oral contraceptive are more prone to develop hypertension in pregnancy, when compared with women whose pressures are unchanged. An important confounding factor is the amount of weight gain and the increasing trend for the use of lower oestrogen content contraceptives and progesterone-only products. There is some evidence of the reverse association, where women who have had a hypertensive pregnancy may be more prone to develop raised blood pressure when taking "the pill".[14] If there is an association, it is weak and should not influence clinical decision making other than the need for careful checking of blood pressure.

Cigarette smoking

Whilst mothers who smoke tend to give birth to smaller babies there is no evidence that they have a higher incidence of pre-eclampsia or any other form of hypertension in pregnancy.

Diabetes mellitus

In the UK Survey of Diabetic Pregnancy (1979–80) the prevalence of pre-eclampsia was 12% in both diabetic women and those developing gestational diabetes.[15] This does represent an excess, but confounding factors including excessive weight gain and its effect on blood pressure may in part explain the findings in women developing gestational diabetes. In patients with pre-existing insulin dependent diabetes mellitus the development of early nephropathy, albeit with hyperfiltrating glomeruli, which will in the short term lower serum creatinine levels, may have influences on blood pressure both in the pregnant and non-pregnant states.[16]

Hydrops fetalis

The prevalence of pre-eclampsia in women with hydrops fetalis has been reported as being between 50% and 70%, this representing a tenfold increased risk.[17]

Hydatidiform mole

Hydatidiform moles substantially increase the risk of pre-eclampsia associated with abnormalities of renal glomerular histology.[17]

Triploidy, fetal malformations and polyhydramnious

It is uncertain whether structural abnormalities of the fetus have much impact on maternal pre-eclampsia.[18] There is an association with polyhydramnios but this may be explained by concurrent diabetes mellitus. Pre-eclampsia is also slightly commoner where the fetus is male.

Practice Point – Risks

- Severe PET is five times more common in twin pregnancies
- There is little evidence for racial differences in the prevalence of PET
- Pre-eclampsia shows some familial concordance
- Diabetes, hydrops and hydatidiform mole all increase the risk of pre-eclampsia

---

Maternal Mortality and Morbidity

In the UK about 8 women per year die as a result of the hypertensive disorders of pregnancy. They tend to be older than average and have more diabetes, hypertension or renal disease.[19]

Maternal morbidity is much less easy to quantify. Strokes are occasionally encountered in late pregnancy, usually related to high blood pressure, and in older women myocardial infarction may occur. They are, however, very rare and related to non-obstetrical causes including familial hypercholesterolaemia and longstanding hypertension.

The syndrome of eclampsia with severe headaches, hyper-reflexia, retinal haemorrhages, cotton wool spots and papilloedema, convulsions and the development of the HELLP syndrome (H = haemolysis, EL = Elevated Liver Enzymes, LP = low platelets) is now rare due to improvements in antenatal care. In the UK eclampsia is reported in 1 in 2000 pregnancies.[20] In 38% of cases there is no prior hypertension or proteinuria. It is three times commoner in women under the age of 20 years and six times commoner in twin pregnancies. In a recent survey 7 out of 383 women (1.85%) died from eclampsia and one other woman was left in a persistent vegetative state. The stillbirth rate after 24 weeks of gestation was 2.2% and the neonatal mortality rate was 3.2%.[20]

Practice Point - Eclampsia

- The UK rate of eclampsia is 1 in 2000 pregnancies
- Eclampsia is three times more common in women < 20 years
- Eclampsia is six times more common in twin pregnancies

Perinatal Mortality

Perinatal mortality rates are gradually improving due to advances in antenatal care, the early detection of hypertension, improved anaesthesia, very early delivery in very high risk mothers and expert neonatal paediatric care.

In 1970 The British Births Survey reported an overall perinatal mortality rate of 21.4 per 1000 pregnancies (Table 2.3), but this figure has almost halved since then.[21] However, these data do demonstrate that mild chronic hypertension, not associated with pre-eclampsia, does not convey excess risk and that the risk of pre-eclampsia is related to its severity.

Table 2.3 Maternal hypertension and perinatal mortality from the British Birth Survey of 1970

	No. of women	Population (%)	No. of perinatal deaths	Perinatal mortality/1000
Normotensive	10 787	63.1	207	19.2
Pre-existing hypertension only	321	1.9	5	15.6
Pre-eclampsia superimposed on pre-existing hypertension	163	1.7	5	30.9
Pre-eclampsia				
mild	2459	16.6	48	19.5
moderate	610	3.5	11	18.1
severe	830	4.8	28	33.7
Remainder	1645	9.4	56	34.2
Total	**16 815**	**100.0**	**360**	**21.4**

These data became available before the widespread use of antihypertensive medication and other important advances in antenatal care. They therefore provide information on the outlook in untreated women with hypertension in pregnancy. Further information on what happens to women with pre-eclampsia with little intervention other than bed-rest and tranquillisers, is provided by a study of 4404 pregnancies between 1960 and 1969 in Finland, all of which were complicated by pre-eclampsia.[22] The perinatal mortality was around 5% in mothers with diastolic blood pressures below 90 mmHg and rose to 25% in those with diastolic pressures of 130 mmHg or more. A similar and perhaps more linear gradient of risk was seen with systolic blood pressure (Figure 2.1).

More up-to-date figures reflecting advances in obstetrical and paediatric care and the more widespread use of antihypertensive drugs may be obtained from the Australian study, which was published in 1997.[4] Using their own inclusive criteria for diagnosing pre-eclampsia, the perinatal mortality rate was 12 per 1000 whilst the more stringent criteria from the USA provide a figure of 38 per 1000 or 3.8%. However, mortality rates now provide an unreliable estimate of the impact of pre-eclampsia due to the improvements in medical care. If the parameter of "small for gestational age" (SGA) is used as an index of perinatal morbidity, then pre-eclampsia is associated with 19% frequency of SGA by the Australian criteria and a 24% frequency by USA criteria.[4] Both

34

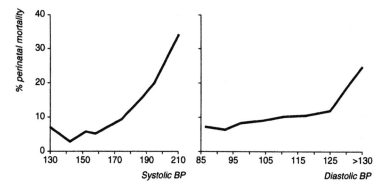

Figure 2.1 Perinatal mortality in pre-eclampsia (1960–1969): study of 4404 pregnancies (from Tervilä *et al.*, 1973,[22] with permission)

of these are high figures and provide a true representation of the hazards of pre-eclampsia in a developed country in the 1990s despite advances in perinatal care.

Perinatal Mortality

- Superimposed pre-eclampsia and severe pre-eclampsia carry the highest risk for the fetus

---

Hypertension in Later Life

There are few reliable long term follow-up studies of the development of later essential hypertension in women with a past history of pre-eclampsia. Two large studies[23, 24] have followed up women who have survived eclampsia for up to 44 years. There was no evidence of an increased prevalence of hypertension compared to that expected from population studies of blood pressure in the community. Several studies reported an excess of later hypertension in women who have had pre-eclampsia mainly after multiparous pregnancies. This finding may, however, reflect a pre-existing tendency to develop essential hypertension, as hypertension in later life was more closely related to mild rather than severe pre-eclampsia. The milder cases will have been those without proteinuria and some of them may have been misclassified. A more recent study from Sweden does, however, contradict this view.[25] After 7 years the frequency of hypertension was 37% (a

35

surprisingly high figure, related possibly to high body weight) in women with non-pre-eclamptic hypertension in pregnancy, 20% in those who had had pre-eclampsia and only 2% (a surprisingly low figure), in volunteer control women of the same age who had had uncomplicated pregnancies. As with the data from America, these figures may be explained in part by methodological considerations and the problems of classification of women with mild hypertension in pregnancy, some of whom may have had essential hypertension. The final verdict is that the long term outlook is uncertain but it would be prudent to carry out periodic checks in all women, and particularly those with a history of hypertension in pregnancy.

References

1 Folkow B, Grimsby G, Thulesius OE. Adaptive structural changes of the vascular walls in hypertension and their relation to the control of the peripheral resistance. *Acta Physiol Scand* 1958;44:252–72.
2 Whelton PK. Epidemiology of hypertension. *Lancet* 1994;334:101–6.
3 Berglund G, Anderson O, Wilhelmson L. Prevalence of primary and secondary hypertension: studies in a random population sample. *Br Med J* 1977;2:554–5.
4 Brown MA, Buddle ML. What's in a name? Problems with the classification of hypertension in pregnancy. *J Hypertens* 1997;15:1049–54.
5 Australasian Society for the Study of Hypertension in Pregnancy. Consensus statement; management of hypertension in pregnancy; executive summary. *Med J Aust* 1993;158:700–2.
6 Davey DA, MacGillivray I. The classification and definition of the hypertensive disorders of pregnancy. *Am J Obstet Gynecol* 1998;158:892–8.
7 National High Blood Pressure Education Program Working Group report on High Blood Pressure in Pregnancy. *Am J Obstet Gynecol* 1990;163:1691–712.
8 Chamberlain G, Elliot P, Howlett B, Masters K. *British Births 1970, Vol. 2, Obstetric Care*. London: Heinemann, 1975.
9 Robillard PY, Hulsey TC. Association of pregnancy-induced-hypertension, pre-eclampsia and eclampsia with duration of sexual cohabitation before conception. *Lancet* 1996;347:619.
10 Thornton JG, Sampson J. Genetics of pre-eclampsia. *Lancet* 1990;336:1319–20.
11 Liston WA, Kilpatrick DG. Is genetic susceptibility to pre-eclampsia conferred by homozygosity for the same single recessive gene in mother and fetus? *Br J Obstet Gynaecol* 1991;98:1079–86.
12 Campbell DM, MacGillivray I, Thompson B. Twin zygosity and pre-eclampsia. *Lancet* 1977;ii:97–101.
13 Page EW, Christianson R. Influence of blood pressure change with and without proteinuria upon outcome of pregnancy. *Am J Obstet Gynecol* 1976; 126:821–33.
14 Khaw K-T, Peart WS. Blood pressure and contraceptive use. *Br Med J* 1982;285:403–7.
15 Lowy C, Beard RW. The British survey of diabetic pregnancies. *Br J Obstet Gynaecol* 1982;89:783–5.
16 White P. Pregnancy complicating diabetes. *Surg Gynaecol Obstet* 1935; 61:324–32.

17 Scott JS. Pregnancy toxaemia associated with hydrops fetalis, hydatidiform mole and hydramnious. *J Obstet Gynaecol Br Emp* 1958;**65**:689–95.
18 MacGillivray I. Hydramnios and pre-eclampsia. *Lancet* 1959;**i**:51–3.
19 Department of Health. *Report on Confidential Enquiries into Maternal Deaths in the United Kingdom 1991–1993*. London: HMSO.
20 Douglas KA, Redman CWG. Eclampsia in the United Kingdom. *Br Med J* 1994;**309**:1395–400.
21 Chamberlain G, Phillip E, Howlett B, Masters K. *British Births 1970, Vol. 2, Obstetric Care*. London: Heinemann, 1978.
22 Tervilä L, Goecke C, Timonen G. Estimation of gestosis of pregnancy (EPH gestosis). *Acta Obstet Gynecol Scand* 1973;**52**:235.
23 Chesney LC, Annitto JE, Cosgrove RA. The remote prognosis of eclamptic women: sixth periodic report. *Am J Obstet Gynecol* 1976;**124**:446–52.
24 Adams EM, MacGillivray I. Long term effect of pre-eclampsia on blood pressure. *Lancet* 1961;**ii**:1373–4.
25 Nissel H, Lintu H, Lunell NO, Mollerstrom G, Pettersson E. Blood pressure and renal function seven years after pregnancy complicated by hypertension. *Br J Obstet Gynaecol* 1995;**102**:876–81.

3 Clinical Assessment and Investigation of the Hypertensive Disorders of Pregnancy

D CHURCHILL AND DG BEEVERS

Introduction

When evaluating mothers suffering from hypertension in pregnancy a combination of assessment methods needs to be employed. In addition, it is important to keep re-testing, if one is to detect early and avert the worst effects of the disease process. Often the trends and changes with time in certain biochemical and haematological variables will foretell of an impending crisis. The same can be said when it comes to assessing the wellbeing of the fetus. One particular measure may be reassuring in the short term, but if the disease process is prolonged then a serial approach to assessing the fetus also needs to be taken.

While obstetricians have several tests with which to assess both the mother and the fetus, it is still important to maintain one's clinical skills and acumen. Therefore we make no apology in this chapter for describing the clinical assessment of the hypertensive patient as well as the other biophysical methods which are used.

When assessing the pre-eclamptic patient certain tests are relied upon more than others. This does not obviate the need to consider the whole patient and some of the more apparently esoteric tests, as the unwary clinician can be drawn into a false sense of security when reliance is placed on only one or two indices. The many varied presentations and complications of pre-eclampsia necessitate a holistic approach.

The Role of the Antenatal Day Assessment Unit

In recent times there have been demands, not least by women themselves, to provide more antenatal care on an outpatient basis or in the community. For the majority of women who have normal pregnancies this is ideal. For women with hypertension and especially pre-eclampsia it is more difficult and sometimes impossible to do this safely. However, where it is safe the development of antenatal day assessment units (ADU) has been helpful to both obstetricians and expectant mothers alike. Day assessment units were established in Scotland well before they migrated south of the border. Audits of their successful activity and specifically in relation to hypertension in pregnancy have been published and are useful texts to refer to when setting up a local unit.[1]

An audit of attendances at the antenatal day assessment unit at Good Hope Hospital for the year 1997 discovered that of the 2107 visits, 12% of patients and 16.3% of patient episodes were for hypertension.

The ADU is helpful for hypertensives in three main ways. First, where there is a doubt about the dependability of the blood pressure readings taken in the antenatal clinic (i.e. is the reading spuriously high due to the white coat effect) a woman can be rested in the ADU, while a series of blood pressure measures can be made, to confirm or refute the suspicion of the white coat effect. This avoids an unnecessary re-visit to the antenatal clinic or worse admission to a ward. Secondly, the ADU is useful for monitoring the effect of newly introduced antihypertensive therapy and finally for more intensive monitoring of the condition of the mother (and fetus) deemed suitable for outpatient management. Each ADU should have midwives skilled in taking blood, interpreting cardiotocographs (CTGs) and able to assess the clinical condition of the hypertensive women. There should be ready access to the ultrasound department for fetal assessment when indicated, but more importantly, there should be immediate access to senior medical staff at all times for guidance and help when managing these difficult cases.

When using the antenatal day unit to manage hypertensive women a fine balance has to be struck between the safety of the mother and fetus and the convenience of outpatient monitoring for the mother. If the condition of the patient is deteriorating (serial biochemical, haematological or biophysical values of both the maternal and fetal condition will provide a good indication of deterioration), there is no substitute for inpatient monitoring of her condition. The complications associated with PET can have an insidious onset and can affect a woman before she realises anything is wrong. There is no home substitute for expert clinical observation and care to detect a worsening clinical condition early and to avert the worst consequences of the disease.

The Clinical Assessment of the Hypertensive Patient

Medical history

It should be remembered that all the causes of hypertension need to be considered when seeing a patient for the first time. The fact that she may be pregnant does not preclude a non-pregnant cause for the hypertension, such as renal disease. Enquiring of a patient's past medical history is just as important as asking if the fetal movements are normal. Any history of renal disease, particularly recurrent urinary infections in early life, should be noted. Hypertension whilst taking the oral contraceptive pill can indicate an individual who is more susceptible to raised blood pressure during pregnancy. A family history of hypertension is another indicator of a person who could have a tendency towards hypertension both in pregnancy and later life. Also, it is common for a woman suffering from pre-eclampsia to relate how her mother or sisters were similarly afflicted during their pregnancies and this should heighten clinical awareness of the possibility of pre-eclampsia.

If patients present *de novo* with hypertension when they book in the first trimester of pregnancy, they will usually be asymptomatic. It is erroneously believed that hypertensives suffer from headaches. Evidence to suggest this is biased by the fact that people complaining of headaches to their physician are more likely to have their blood pressure measured, than are patients with other symptomatology. It is only when end organ damage as a result of hypertension has started that patients begin to complain of symptoms. Dyspnoea, orthopnoea and paroxysmal nocturnal dyspnoea are signs of heart failure. Fatigue, vomiting and/or oedema may indicate renal damage, and visual disturbances may indicate compromise of the cerebral circulation. For women of reproductive age who are discovered to be hypertensive these symptoms are rare findings, as end organ damage is unlikely to have started.

For women who develop hypertension after 20 weeks' gestation, the primary diagnosis of pre-eclampsia needs more active consideration. The history taken from these women should include all of the above features but in addition one needs to enquire for any symptoms which appear to be specific to pre-eclampsia. Headache is a frequent and often early finding in affected individuals. It is often sited in the frontal region of the head and behind the eyes. It is a nagging, dull pain, not relieved by simple analgesics and will often only partially respond to strong painkillers. Some women merely describe having a "muzzy" head. This too should be considered as a serious symptom. A general feeling of puffiness is another symptom, which is often expressed by these patients and relates to an element of generalised oedema. Swelling of the ankles is a common finding in up to 70% of all pregnant women, but swelling of the fingers and face is a more significant finding.

Visual disturbances, spots in front of the eyes or floating bodies passing across the field of vision are another symptom associated with pre-eclampsia and a sign of worsening disease, as are the symptoms of nausea and vomiting. Swelling of the liver from an increase in tissue fluid causes epigastric or right hypochondrial pain as the expansion stretches the liver capsule. Other more severe symptoms, such as dyspnoea, haemoptysis, chest pain etc., indicate very severe disease with multisystem involvement.

Medical History

- Symptoms: headaches, visual disturbances, flushing, dyspnoea, chest pain, nausea and vomiting
- Past history: previous complicated pregnancies, past contraceptive complications, past renal disease or recurrent urinary tract infections
- Family history: pregnancy outcome for mother and sisters
- Social history: social circumstances, single or supported, smoking, alcohol

---

Physical examination

The physical examination of a hypertensive pregnant woman needs to be comprehensive. All systems, cardiovascular, respiratory, gastrointestinal/abdominal and nervous need careful attention. For example, a heart murmur heard all over the praecordium and at the back of the thorax, along with radiofemoral delay in the transmission of the pulse from the heart downstream to the femoral arteries, indicate coarctation of the aorta. Heart murmurs of any significance need assessment by a cardiologist who may order an echocardiogram.

Renal artery bruits in the abdomen can indicate stenosis of these arteries, which in young women may be due to fibromuscular dysplasia. Features of corticosteroid excess may point to Cushing's disease, although abdominal striae etc. are features found in normal pregnancies at later gestations. When examining the abdomen, tenderness over the renal angles may indicate pyelonephritis or other chronic infection.

Fundoscopy should be carried out in all hypertensive patients, especially those suffering from pre-eclampsia. Hypertensive retinopathy may be detected in all of its forms, from the very mild grade I, arteriovenous nipping and silver wiring, to the severe grade III with papilloedema. The latter, although a rare finding, indicates severe disease, with treatment required urgently. If the blood pressure is not controlled in this situation, then cerebrovascular accidents are a very real risk. In the absence of severe hypertension, other causes of raised intracranial pressure should be considered.

Patients with severe pre-eclampsia may show signs of neural irritability. Hyperreflexia can often be demonstrated in normal pregnancy but the presence of more than one beat of clonus is always a pathological finding, especially in association with pre-eclampsia. It may signify that the patient is close to suffering an eclamptic fit.

Women with pre-eclampsia may also exhibit various other signs relating to the many varied presentations of the syndrome. An enlarged liver stretching the capsule causes tenderness in the right hypochondrium.

A recent American review of high order multiple pregnancies, triplets and quads found that atypical presentations of the pre-eclampsia syndrome such as HELLP (haemolysis, elevated liver enzymes and low platelets) predominated in these pregnancies.[2] Hypertension was often not the presenting sign and abnormal laboratory values were discovered more frequently than a rise in BP.

Practice Point – Physical Examination

- Cardiovascular: blood pressure, heart sounds, peripheral pulses
- Respiratory: auscultate for pulmonary oedema in severe PET
- Abdominal: palpate for hepatic tenderness. Assess the consistency of the uterus, its size as well as the presentation and lie of the fetus
- Reflexes: clonus
- Fundoscopy: inspect each retina for retinopathy grades I–III

Haematological and Biochemical Investigations in the Mother

Both newly diagnosed hypertensives in early pregnancy and pre-eclamptics in later pregnancy need thoroughly investigating. These investigations will differ slightly depending upon the diagnostic priorities. In early pregnancy identifying any underlying cause for hypertension is important, whereas after 20 weeks' gestation the investigations will be tailored to making the diagnosis and determining the severity of pre-eclampsia. There will, however, be a great deal of overlap between the two situations and their investigation will be considered in tandem.

Trends and changes in the levels of serum and blood indicators are often more important than the absolute levels themselves. It is our practice and recommendation that the measurements made are entered on a flow sheet. Abnormal trends can be readily identified early in the course of the disease, warning the clinician of an impending crisis.

Practice Point – Measurement

- The use of flow charts makes the identification of adverse trends in multiple parameters more readily identifiable and thus gives a better warning of an impending crisis

---

Full blood count

A full blood count is almost carried out unthinkingly these days, however it can yield vital information when investigating the hypertensive pregnant woman. Anaemia will increase the heart rate and cardiac output (which in pregnant women is already raised), thus exacerbating the hypertension. Therefore in general terms correcting the anaemia is important in helping to improve the general wellbeing of the woman and to reduce the physiological tendency to increase the underlying levels of blood pressure. The majority of cases of true anaemia in pregnancy are due to a deficiency of iron, which can be readily corrected with oral supplementation. Alternatively, a fall in the haemoglobin may be due to haemolysis and a blood film may reveal damaged red blood cells in the maternal circulation, prompting further consideration of the HELLP syndrome as a possible diagnosis. Erythroblasts may rarely be detected if the haemolysis has been going on for some period of time.

A relatively high haemoglobin for pregnancy may indicate haemoconcentration, which can be confirmed by examining the haematocrit. A raised haematocrit will signify a depletion of the intravascular blood volume, with serum leaking out into the extravascular spaces. This is pathognomonic of pre-eclampsia and can indicate worsening disease.[3]

It is important to monitor the platelet count in pre-eclampsia. Large studies estimate that approximately 20% of patients with pre-eclampsia develop a mild thrombocytopenia ($< 150 \times 10^9$/l).[4] An acute 20–30% fall in the platelet count in successive measurements is a significant finding, indicating severe disease and necessitates careful future monitoring of the platelet count. Once the count falls below 100×10^9/l the slide will usually continue, and while this level does not impair coagulation, levels below 50×10^9/l are more critical. The haematologists will need to be informed of such a situation and be requested to have pooled platelets ready for transfusion should an emergency operative delivery be required. Thrombocytopenia caused by pre-eclampsia results from a reduction in the platelet lifespan from 9 to 5 days and an increased level of platelet activation. These platelets then adhere to the sites of endothelial cell damage, which in the case of PET is thought to be occurring in the uteroplacental vasculature. There is evidence to show that the effect upon platelets in PET is due to a relative imbalance between thromboxane and prostacyclin. Thromboxane is itself a powerful vasoconstrictor and platelet aggregator.

Urea, creatinine, and electrolytes

These measurements are as ubiquitous as the full blood count, but also provide valuable information about the condition of the patient. In normal pregnancy the urea and creatinine should be at the lower end of the normal range. A urea in the upper end of this range is abnormal and indicates an impaired renal function.[5] Normal ranges for these indices in pregnancy are available and should be consulted when considering biochemical results.[6] The creatinine rises only in severe cases of renal failure, as do derangements of the levels of sodium and potassium. In the vast majority of cases there will be no significant changes in the levels of creatinine, sodium, or potassium. These indices are unfortunately insensitive and, when they are found to be abnormal, the pre-eclampsia and hence renal damage is usually at an advanced stage. Abnormally high levels of urea and creatinine for pregnancy indicate a very significant degree of renal compromise. In these situations the clinician needs to be watchful, especially when giving fluids, as the risk of iatrogenic fluid overload is enhanced in patients with renal impairment, especially by the careless administration of intravenous crystalloids and colloids.

Uric acid

This is probably the most utilised investigation for assessing the severity of pre-eclampsia. Like a conditioned reflex, obstetricians request the level of uric acid before any of the other investigations in PET. Of all the investigations carried out, it has generally been found to be useful when differentiating pre-eclampsia from chronic hypertension, when it is usually within the normal range. It is also useful prognostically, as for any given level of blood pressure the higher the level of urate, the greater the perinatal mortality.[7] A raised uric acid in the maternal blood results from tissue ischaemia and reduced renal clearance. Uric acid is actively excreted by the distal convoluted tubule of the kidney, after being reabsorbed through the proximal tubule. Damage to the distal tubule in pre-eclampsia means that urate is not excreted and so remains in the circulation.[8] A raised serum urate can be the forerunner of the proteinuria and it is prudent not to ignore a high uric acid level in any woman with raised blood pressure, even in the absence of any other signs of the disease. They invariably do develop the full syndrome, although the timescale over which this occurs is variable.

While uric acid is an important test to use when assessing the condition of a pre-eclamptic patient, it should not be exclusively relied upon. Renal function may be relatively unaffected and yet the patient found to be severely ill with one of the other associated syndrome complexes, such as HELLP.

Liver function studies

A raised alkaline phosphatase is commonly found in late pregnancy. Isoenzyme studies reveal this to be mainly placental in origin, so in isolation this is not necessarily a sign of liver damage. When other enzymes are raised, such as alanine aminotransferase, aspartate aminotransferase or gamma glutamyl transferase, then hepatocellular damage is undoubtedly occurring. This can be a very serious situation heralding the onset of the HELLP syndrome. If ongoing damage is ignored it could lead to coagulopathies developing at a very rapid rate. In cases where liver damage is occurring the condition of the patient needs close monitoring. If there are signs of accelerating hepatic damage immediate delivery of the fetus is the only course of action. The liver will then spontaneously recover its full function in time. If it is ignored the liver failure may result in the development of serious multisystem disorders, such as the hepatorenal syndrome, and thus make the treatment of the patient more difficult. In many women the abnormalities in the liver function tests will be static or only deteriorating very slowly. These patients can be managed conservatively, although regular serum liver function testing, two to three times a week, will be necessary to follow the course of the disease process. Once again the normal ranges for liver function tests in pregnancy are different from the non-pregnant state. Interpretation of these investigations in pre-eclamptic patients should be carried out in comparison with ranges set for normal pregnancies.[9]

Criteria for the Diagnosis of the HELLP Syndrome

- Haemolysis–raised lactate dehydrogenase (LDH) and evidence of red cell destruction on a peripheral blood film
- Elevated liver enzymes aspartate and alanine aminotransferases
- Low platelets $< 150 \times 10^9/l$

Twenty-four hour urinary output of total protein

While the definition of pre-eclampsia can be made using dipstix analysis of the urine, it is advisable to assess the quantity of protein loss through the kidneys during a 24 hour period with a urine collection.[10] Significant proteinuria in early pregnancy, associated with chronic hypertension, indicates the possibility of an underlying nephritis. These patients need to be followed up after pregnancy by the appropriate renal specialist. A renal biopsy may be necessary to define the exact nature of the renal pathology (see Chapter 8).

A large 24 hour urinary protein loss is another marker of the severity of the patient's condition. A review of 444 pregnancies showed that those women who were losing greater than 300 mg of protein in their urine during a 24 hour period, were at a significantly increased risk of a poor perinatal outcome.[11] The pathophysiological change of glomerular endotheliosis causes increased leakage of protein into the urine. The amount of leakage may be reflected in a low level of serum albumin and total protein. This then alters the intravascular oncotic pressure and causes the patient to suffer from generalised oedema. A low serum protein level is particularly problematic for those treating acutely ill pre-eclamptic patients. Correct fluid management is critical for the wellbeing of these patients.

The vascular endothelial damage causes leakage of serum protein and fluid into the extracellular spaces. In the presence of low serum protein levels, administering high volumes of crystalloids and colloids intravenously will worsen the oedema and can cause pulmonary oedema. This could then lead to adult respiratory distress syndrome (ARDS) if it is not recognised early and treated promptly. A significant number of maternal deaths are recorded every triennium from this particular condition, usually in association with pre-eclampsia.

Equally, replacing protein intravenously while it is being lost through the kidneys tends to have little beneficial effect. It is usually better to wait until the protein loss has stopped or diminished to very low levels, before administering additional protein as only then will it remain in the circulation, raising the plasma oncotic pressure and thus draw in fluid from the extracellular spaces. Only rarely may it be necessary to give intravenous albumin when the loss is heavy through the kidneys. The risk is that the albumin will leak out through the damaged endothelium into

47

the extracellular spaces, worsening the tissue oedema. If the urinary output is at such a low level that it threatens acute renal failure, it is more usual to stimulate a diuresis with loop diuretics. This therefore avoids the risk of pushing more fluid into the wrong tissue compartment, creating more problems for these critically ill patients.

While a 24 hour urine collection for total protein is important when making a diagnosis of pre-eclampsia, serial measurements made in cases of severe pre-eclampsia managed conservatively are of little prognostic value. In such women the amount of protein lost will continue to increase at variable rates and a slower rate of increase should not be interpreted as less severe disease.[12]

Practice Point – Maternal Investigations

- Full blood count: haemoglobin, haematocrit, platelet count and blood film if there is any evidence of haemolysis
- Biochemistry: urea, creatinine, electrolytes, and uric acid, liver function tests
- 24 hour urine save: total protein assessment ± catecholamines
- Others: ANA, anti-cardiolipin, lupus anticoagulant, for early onset PET, i.e. < 32 weeks

---

Minimum Standards for Maternal Monitoring in Patients with Pre-eclampsia and Ongoing Pregnancies

- 4 hourly blood pressure monitoring
- Daily urine analysis for the level of protein loss (dipstix testing will suffice)
- Twice weekly platelet count and serum uric acid measurement
- Weekly assessment of the liver function

Additional Investigations

Phaeochromocytoma

While overall phaeochromocytoma is a rare cause of hypertension, accounting for 0.5% of all patients with high blood pressure, there are reports of its discovery during pregnancy.[13, 14] Hypertension is sustained in about half of the patients with this condition but all sufferers tend to exhibit episodic rises in blood pressure, often to extremely high levels. Symptoms complained of include sudden pounding headaches, palpitations, sweating and tremors. Exercise, anxiety, bowel movements and micturition can trigger paroxysmal attacks. During these attacks the patient may exhibit extreme pallor and their skin become mottled and afterwards they become weak and exhausted. Because of its seriousness, it is important to detect this condition promptly. A 24 hour urine collection for vanillylmandelic acid (VMA) or the other metabolites of adrenaline and noradrenaline should be performed. Once the diagnosis is made biochemically, then a search for the source of the excess of adrenaline and noradrenaline should begin. The adrenal glands and sympathetic chain are the most likely sites. It is uncommon for the tumour to be palpable in the abdomen and imaging of these areas with ultrasound or computed tomography (CT) is usually needed.[15] Once the tumour has been detected, the treatment of choice is to remove it surgically. However, this may not be possible during the pregnancy and one may wish to wait for fetal lung maturity before ending the pregnancy and proceeding with a surgical cure. In these very rare instances it may be possible to control the hypertension with alpha- and beta-blockade to gain valuable time. In any event specialist help will be required (see Chapter 8).

Anti-phospholipid syndrome

Anti-phospholipid syndrome is more commonly associated with early pregnancy loss but has also been found in conjunction with early onset pre-eclampsia, at between 25 and 30 weeks' gestation.[16, 17] In pregnancies complicated by early disease, it is worthwhile testing patients' sera for anti-nuclear antibodies as a general screen before proceeding to look for lupus anticoagulant and anti-phospholipid antibodies, including the anti-cardiolipin antibodies. These conditions predispose to excessive platelet consumption and thrombosis, causing placental ischaemia and infarction.[18, 19] Low dose aspirin therapy will help to prevent some of the platelet consumption and thus placental ischaemia; and theoretically may improve the overall prognosis. The same groups of conditions are worth considering in women who have suffered from recurrent abortions or had children with severe intrauterine growth retardation. These women are also prone to thromboembolism, and in women who have additional risk factors it may be worth considering adding subcutaneous heparin to the therapeutic regimen partly as a prophylactic measure against deep vein thrombosis.

> ### Practice Point – Management
>
> - The changes and rates of change in the levels of the various indices being used to monitor the disease process are often more important than the absolute levels themselves

Maternal Complications of Pre-eclampsia

Most of the severe complications of pre-eclampsia are thankfully rare. However, when they do occur they can have profound and serious consequences for the mother and the whole family if they result in long term morbidity. The most common and best known complication is eclampsia. If treated appropriately and promptly the mother will make a full and uncomplicated recovery. If, however, the seizure is associated with a cerebrovascular accident, either a haemorrhage or infarct, long term neurological damage can result. These complications can take the form of a sensory motor stroke or cortical blindness. However, not all blindness is due to cortical problems. Retinal detachment and oedema are also recognised complications and equally need effective treatment to avoid adverse long term sequelae.

As well as the HELLP syndrome, the coagulation system can be affected by disseminated intravascular coagulation (DIC) and microangiopathic haemolysis. Liver damage in itself, such as capsule rupture or hepatic infarction, can reduce the capacity of the liver to produce clotting factors, as well as carry out its other vital metabolic functions.

Acute tubular necrosis and unspecified renal failure is another of the many complications. Fortunately the renal function improves after delivery, when the disease process is halted. Very occasionally some women need renal dialysis but these unlucky few usually recover after a few weeks of treatment.

Pulmonary oedema and ARDS are complications, which often have an iatrogenic basis. Poor fluid management and fluid overload of only minor degrees will lead to these complications. The endothelial damage in the lung causes the ready leakage of fluid into the interstitial spaces. Laryngeal oedema can also result in airways obstruction and cause problems for the anaesthetists when trying to intubate a severely ill pre-eclamptic. Patients with pre-eclampsia need an experienced anaesthetist in attendance, especially if a general anaesthetic is being administered.

Maternal Complications

- Eclampsia
- Cerebrovascular accidents
- Myocardial infarction
- Renal failure
- Disseminated intravascular coagulation
- Retinal detachment
- HELLP
- Adult respiratory distress syndrome

Fetal Assessment

Estimation of fetal size

Hypertensive disease, especially pre-eclampsia, causes intra-uterine growth restriction/retardation (IUGR); and once the diagnosis of PET is made, a scan should be requested to estimate the size of the fetus. Clinical assessment of fetal growth, usually by measuring the symphysiofundal height, is inaccurate and should not be relied upon to assess the growth of the fetus in the high-risk pregnancy. Even when a tape measure is used the intra- and interobserver errors are great and real time ultrasound scanning is a more accurate method of measuring the fetal growth pattern.[20] The two most important scan measures are the head and abdominal circumferences (HC and AC) (Figures 3.1, 3.2). Often the abdominal circumference (AC) is the first measure to fall from its intended growth curve. A fetus chronically starved of oxygen and nutrients is unable to lay down fat and glycogen stores in the liver, as it is using these substrates for its own energy requirements. The growth of the head is preserved as oxygenated blood is shunted to the vital organs–the brain, adrenals, and heart. Later the growth of the head will be affected, falling off its intended curve, although by the time this occurs the fetus has usually suffered a very significant hypoxaemic insult. Once discovered, a growth-restricted fetus starved of oxygen needs further assessment, both ultrasonically and by examining the fetal heart rate.

51

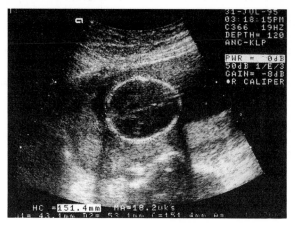

Figure 3.1   An ultrasound image of a normal fetal head circumference.

Biophysical profile

The biophysical profile (BPP) is a dynamic method of observing fetal behaviour over a period of time which has been found to correlate with its general wellbeing. There are five components to the profile: these are, fetal movements, fetal tone, fetal breathing movements, the liquor volume and fetal heart rate assessment. It

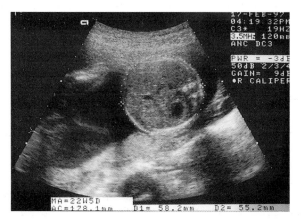

Figure 3.2   An ultrasound image of a normal fetal abdominal circumference.

Table 3.1   Fetal biophysical profile scoring system.

Variable	Score 0	Score 2
Cardiotocography	No accelerations	Normal accelerations
Fetal breathing	<30 s breathing	At least 30 s of sustained breathing in 30 min
Fetal movements	<3 movements	3 or more gross body movements in 30 min
Fetal tone	No movements	At least one motion of limb flexion to extension and back
Amniotic fluid volume	<1 cm² fluid	A pocket of fluid at least 2 cm in depth

has been shown experimentally in animals that loss of these biophysical variables occurs with increasing hypoxaemia.[21] Therefore the test has some scientific credence. A scoring system has been applied to the BPP, with a normal feature scoring 2 and the absence of a feature not scoring at all (see Table 3.1).[22] A score out of 10 is given, and in conjunction with the clinical situation an informed management plan can be developed for the rest of the pregnancy. Generally, a BPP score of 8 or 10 is a reassuring finding.

The problem with the biophysical profile score as it stands is that each component is given the same clinical importance. However the most important single feature of the BPP is the liquor volume and oligo- or anhydramnios is a seriously worrying finding even when the other components of the profile are present. In addition to the liquor volume, fetal breathing movements seem to be a sensitive indicator of cerebral hypoxaemia.[23]

Another difficulty with the BPP is that it is time consuming. The natural cyclical activity of the fetus means that to comment with surety that a particular feature of fetal activity is absent needs at least a 40 minute examination, although the mean time quoted to perform a full BPP in a population study is 15 minutes. Randomised studies of BPP testing have been performed and a meta-analysis showed no support for the use of the BPP.[24] However, the number of studies and patients entered into these trials are small and unlikely to have shown any benefit in terms of significant outcome measures such as mortality. Much of the evidence for the BPP has come from large open prospective studies. Pregnancies monitored with the BPP showed a perinatal mortality within one week of a normal BPP to be 0.7 per 1000, which was far superior to the cardiotocograph as a predictor of perinatal outcome.[21] While the figures are impressive, comparative data with less extensive monitoring protocols was not made and so the necessity of a full BPP on every occasion is questionable.

Others have suggested an abbreviated biophysical profile, using heart rate testing and liquor volume in the first instance, before moving on to a full biophysical profile in those fetuses exhibiting abnormal features.[25] There is outcome evidence reported showing that two stage testing in this way is just as successful in assessing the fetal wellbeing as the more formal, full BPP.

Whichever way fetal wellbeing is assessed, it is important that it is carried out thoroughly and efficiently, by well-trained observers. If the full BPP is used then the time taken over the examination should be noted, to prevent the unwary obstetrician from acting on a low score, which may simply be due to the natural sleep–wake cycle of the fetus. Despite its limitations, testing fetal wellbeing with ultrasound is helpful in giving the obstetrician an overall view of the pregnancy, especially in cases complicated by hypertension, pre-eclampsia, IUGR or a combination of all these three.

Cardiotocography

This method of assessing fetal health is more immediate, although some degree of reassurance for the next 48 hours can be gained from a normal tracing (Figure 3.3). An assessment of a cardiotocograph should include an examination of the baseline fetal heart rate, the variability about the baseline and accelerations. A normal fetal heart rate (FHR) pattern consists of a baseline between 110 and 150 beats per minute (bpm), periodic accelerations greater than 15 bpm over and above the baseline for a total of 15 seconds or more; and a variability about the baseline of between 5 and 15 bpm (Figure 3.4). As gestational age increases the baseline decreases; some post-term pregnancies have baselines between 100 and 110 bpm, and the number of accelerations increases. In normal circumstances baseline variability increases with periods of fetal activity.[26]

The absence of accelerations in a 45 minute period is highly suspicious of "fetal distress", in the absence of any other cause, such as anti-hypertensive medication where high doses of labetalol or nifedipine may result in a steal effect on the uteroplacental circulation.

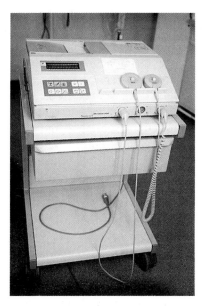

Figure 3.3 Oxford Instruments 800 meridian fetal heart monitor. This model has the ability to monitor twin pregnancies.

Decelerations are generally pathological. The nadir of early or type 1 decelerations does not fall more than 40 beats below the baseline FHR. They also begin and end with the uterine contraction cycle. Deeper falls in the FHR are termed variable decelerations and are most commonly found in association with cord entanglement. A deceleration which begins at the end of a contraction cycle and lasts for 30 seconds or more after cessation of the contraction is called late or type 2 deceleration. When associated with a reduction in baseline variability, these decelerations are highly suggestive of a decrease in cerebral oxygenation.[27] Decelerations in the fetal heart in the antenatal period are often observed without any uterine activity being registered by the tocograph. In these circumstances it is necessary for the clinician to examine the whole case and possibly perform other assessments of fetal wellbeing before forming a judgement about the cause of such FHR abnormalities.

Abnormal FHR patterns are more likely to be found in pregnancies where the placental circulation is compromised. Pre-

55

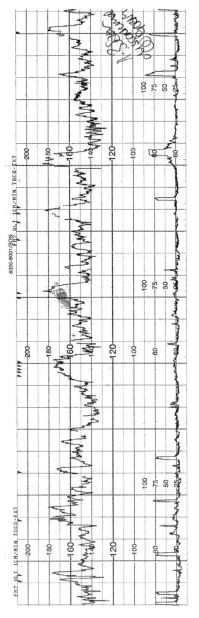

Figure 3.4 A cardiotocograph showing an entirely normal fetal heart rate pattern.

eclampsia being caused by placental ischaemia itself is likely to be associated with such patterns. However, the thoughtful clinician must also remember that anti-hypertensive treatment can adversely affect the uteroplacental circulation and FHR.

More recently, computerised assessment of the antenatal fetal heart rate has been developed and the "Oxford" system is now widely used (Figure 3.5). This system provides a more sophisticated analysis of the fetal heart rate, taking into account its natural cycle over a 40 minute period. Each component is defined slightly differently. For example, the baseline is taken as the mean fetal heart rate in the absence of fetal movement, i.e. during a "low episode". The short term variability is a measure of the average of sequential 1/16th minute pulse interval differences over a period of 3.75 milliseconds. The full details of the analytical techniques are beyond the scope of this book. If the reader requires more information, the reports by Professor Dawes are recommended reading for the technically minded.[28, 29] The system has been tested on tens of thousands of patients and is constantly updated. Another

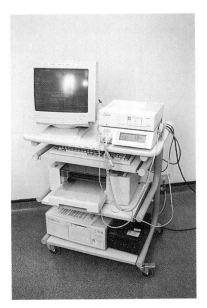

Figure 3.5 Oxford Instruments System 8002 Objective CTG analysis system. This system stores the recording electronically for future reference.

advantage is that the computer produces a report of the analysis (Figure 3.6), thus largely removing the intra- and interobserver variation from the assessment. In addition, work has been produced giving the risks of fetal hypoxia at various levels of short term variation, which is measured in milliseconds (Table 3.2). This system has been a great advance in the cardiotocographic assessment of the high-risk fetus.

In the absence of computerised analysis the printout of the FHR pattern must be analysed carefully. The recording should be of sufficient duration, at least 45 minutes in the absence of any acceleration in the first 20 minutes of the tracing. The observer should classify the characteristics of each component. When the assessment of the pattern is complete the findings should be assessed in conjunction with the whole clinical picture before any management decisions are taken. Assessing the FHR pattern in isolation will risk both too early intervention and delivery of normal fetuses on the one hand, or false reassurance in ill fetuses when other parameters such as Doppler waveforms may be abnormal.

Doppler ultrasound (Figure 3.7)

Evidence has shown that in high-risk pregnancies Doppler ultrasound of the umbilical artery reduces perinatal mortality. The odds of perinatal death are reduced by 38% (95% confidence intervals 15%–55%).[30] Conditions like pre-eclampsia lend themselves well to assessment using Doppler ultrasound because their origins lie within the vasculature of the placenta. Pre-eclamptic pregnancies, especially those complicated by fetal growth restriction, will show higher impedance to flow through the placenta. In severe cases this will result in the loss or reversal of flow in the diastolic phase of the cardiac cycle. These fetuses are at very high risk of hypoxaemia and, when this is prolonged, acidaemia. The correlation between absent or reversed end diastolic flow, placental failure and fetal hypoxaemia is strong and warrants immediate plans to increase surveillance of the fetus with the biophysical methods previously described.[31] Although in many situations immediate delivery of the fetus will be appropriate, this is not necessary in all instances.

Problems remain over the semi-quantitative measures of resistance; the pulsatility index, resistance index, and systolic/diastolic ratio. Clinical outcome in relation to high values is still clouded

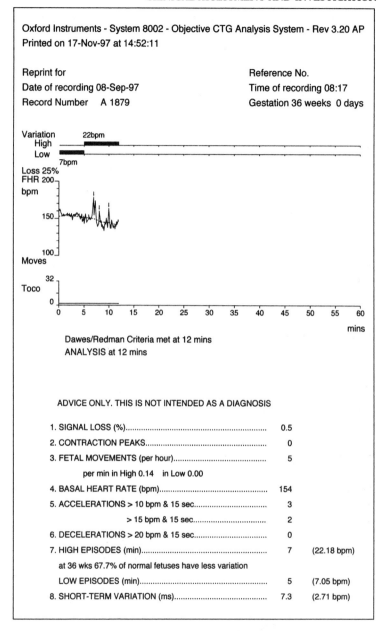

Figure 3.6 A report from the System 8002. The analysis of the fetal heart rate pattern shows a healthy fetus.

Table 3.2   The short term variability measured in milliseconds correlated with the likelihood of fetal acidaemia in percentages.

Short term variability in ms	Percentage likelihood of metabolic acidaemia
>4	0
3.5–4	8
3.0–3.5	29
2.5–3.0	33
<2.5	72

with uncertainty, and based upon current evidence it would be inappropriate to decide the course of a pregnancy on the basis of a raised reading from these measures.[32] An area where they may prove useful is in studying the trend over time. A rising level of resistance as a pregnancy proceeds may indicate ongoing placental

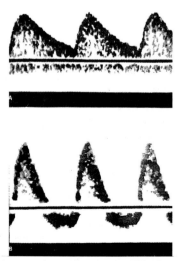

Figure 3.7   Doppler waveforms from an umbilical artery. The upper plate shows a normal pattern. The lower plate shows an abnormal waveform with reversed flow in the diastolic phase of the cardiac cycle.

damage and may be more significant than a level which falls with gestation.

Another area of research being undertaken utilising Doppler ultrasound is fetal regional blood flow studies. With colour flow mapping available on many machines it is relatively easy to examine the flow in the cerebral circulation, aorta, ductus arteriosus, renal vessels etc.[33] While there is some evidence that studying regional blood flow in the fetus may be useful, it has yet to enter mainstream clinical practice.

From the evidence of the randomised trials the value of Doppler ultrasound reducing perinatal mortality in high-risk pregnancies seems proven (Figure 3.8). The assessment of a fetus of a hypertensive pregnancy, especially one where the mother has pre-eclampsia, will add valuable information to the clinical picture and allow a more accurate assessment of fetal wellbeing.

Comparisons and outcomes
Doppler ultrasound in high-risk pregnancies

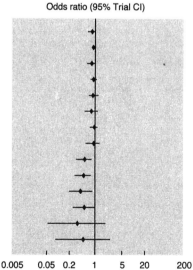

Figure 3.8   A meta-analysis of trials of Doppler ultrasound in high-risk pregnancies, pooling the results of the outcome measures. Perinatal deaths and stillbirths are reduced when Doppler is used to assess pregnancies.

Practice Point–Fetal Assessment

- Ultrasound estimation of fetal size: head and abdominal circumferences and the ratio between the two
- Biophysical profile: fetal movement, tone, breathing movements and liquor volume + fetal heart rate assessment (see below)
- Cardiotocography: standard or computerised
- Doppler ultrasound: umbilical arteries, uterine arteries, ± fetal regional studies
- Others: amniocentesis, fetal blood sampling

Minimum Standards for Fetal Monitoring in Patients with Pre-eclampsia and On-going Pregnancies

- Daily cardiotocography–if computerised CTGs are used a synoptic may be useful each week
- Ultrasound assessment of the fetal weight and growth profile at 2 weekly intervals
- Twice weekly ultrasound assessment for liquor volume
- Twice weekly umbilical artery Doppler ultrasound assessment

---

Summary

When a mother is diagnosed as suffering from a hypertensive disease in pregnancy a full assessment of the whole pregnancy is required. In early pregnancy, prior to 20 weeks' gestation, a search for endocrine and renal causes of the hypertension should be undertaken. The onset of hypertension after 20 weeks' gestation should alert the clinician to the possibility of pre-eclampsia. When this diagnosis is made, serial haematological and biochemical measurements will need to be carried out on the mother. Often the clinical condition may be stable, when the haematological and biochemical indices are severely deranged. The fetus also needs to be very carefully monitored in women suffering from pre-eclampsia. They too can be affected by the placental ischaemia, resulting in growth restriction and chronic hypoxia. In fetuses considered to be at risk the primary assessment should be to estimate the fetus size and liquor volume ultrasonically as well as carry out umbilical artery Doppler waveform analysis. In addition, a cardiotocograph, preferably of the computerised variety, should be carried out. If any of these parameters gives cause for concern, the fetus should either undergo full biophysical testing, with possibly regional Doppler blood flow studies, or if the abnormality is sufficiently concerning, i.e. severe heart rate abnormalities on the CTG, be delivered. Ultimately delivery is the only cure for pre-eclampsia and it is important not to over-monitor the condition or the fetus and lose sight of the overall clinical picture.

References

1 Walker JJ. The management of mild/moderate hypertension in pregnancy–the use of antenatal day care assessment. In: Walker JJ, Gant NF, eds. *Hypertension in pregnancy.* London: Chapman & Hall, 1997.

2 Hardardottir H, Kelly K, Bork MD et al. Atypical presentation of pre-eclampsia in high-order multifetal gestations. *Obstet Gynecol* 1996;87:370–4.

3 Sibai BM. Eclampsia. In: Birkenhager WH, Reid JL, eds. *Handbook of hypertension, Vol. 10, Hypertension in pregnancy.* Amsterdam: Elsevier, 1988.

4 Redman CWG, Bonnar J, Beilin L. Early platelet consumption in pre-eclampsia. *Br Med J* 1978;1:467–9.

5 Wichman K, Ryden G. Blood pressure and renal function during normal pregnancy. *Acta Obstet Gynecol Scand* 1986;65:561–6.

6 Ramsay MM, James DK, Steer PJ, Weiner CP, Gonik B. *Normal values in pregnancy.* London: WB Saunders, 1996.

7 Hunt HF, Patterson WB, Nicodemus RE. Placental infarction and eclampsia. *Am J Clin Pathol* 1940;10:319.

8 Redman CWG, Bonnar J. Plasma urate changes in pre-eclampsia. *Br Med J* 1978;I:1484–5.

9 Girling JC, Dow E, Smith JH. Liver function tests in pre-eclampsia: importance of comparison with a reference range derived for normal pregnancy. *Br J Obstet Gynaecol* 1997;104:246–50.

10 Kuo VS, Koumantakis G, Gallery EDM. Proteinuria and its assessment in normal and hypertensive pregnancy. *Am J Obstet Gynecol* 1992;167:723–8.

11 Ferrazani S, Caruso A, De Carolis S, Vercillo Martino I, Mancuso S. Proteinuria and outcome of 444 pregnancies complicated by hypertension. *Am J Obstet Gynecol* 1990;162:366–71.

12 Schiff E, Friedman SA, Kao L, Sibai BM. The importance of urinary protein excretion during conservative management of severe pre-eclampsia. *Am J Obstet Gynecol* 1996;175:1313–16.

13 Lau P, Permezel M, Dawson P et al. Phaeochromocytoma in pregnancy. *Aust NZ J Obstet Gynecol* 1996;36:472–6.

14 Atan A, Yildiz M, Aydoganli L, Gullu I, Akalin Z. Phaeochromocytoma in pregnancy: a case report. *Int Urol Nephrol* 1996;28:11–13.

15 Heikkinen AM, Alhava E, Haring P, Suonio S, Saarikoski S. Phaeochromocytoma in pregnancy. *Ann Chir Gynaecol* 1994;83:69–72.

16 Oshiro BT, Silver RM, Scott JR, Yu H, Branch W. Antiphospholipid antibodies and fetal death. *Obstet Gynecol* 1996;87:489–93.

17 Branch DW, Andres R, Digre KB, Rote NS, Scott JR. The association of antiphospholipid antibodies with pre-eclampsia *Obstet Gynecol* 1989;73:541–5.

18 Alsulyman OM, Castro MA, Zuckerman E, McGehee W, Murphy Goodwin T. Pre-eclampsia and liver infarction in early pregnancy associated with the antiphospholipid syndrome. *Obstet Gynecol* 1996;88:644–6.

19 Arnout J, Spitz B, van Assche A, Vermylen J. The antiphospholipid syndrome and pregnancy. *Hyperten Preg* 1995;14:147–78.
20 Whittle MJ. Fetal growth. In: Dewsbury K, Meire H, Cosgrove D, eds. *Ultrasound in obstetrics and gynaecology.* London: Churchill Livingstone, 1994.
21 Manning FA. Dynamic ultrasound based fetal assessment: the fetal biophysical score. *Clin Obstet Gynaecol* 1995;38:26–44.
22 Manning FA, Platt L, Sipos L. Antepartum fetal evaluation. Development of a fetal biophysical profile. *Am J Obstet Gynecol* 1980;136:787–95.
23 Walkinshaw SA. Biophysical profiles. *Curr Obstet Gynecol* 1977;7:74–81.
24 Alfrevic Z, Neilson JP. Biophysical profile for fetal assessment in high risk pregnancy. In: Enkin MW, Keirse M, Renfrew M, Neilson JP, eds. *Pregnancy and childbirth module of the Cochrane database of systematic reviews.* Cochrane Library. The Cochrane Collaboration Issue 3, Oxford Update.
25 Mills MS, James DK, Slade S. Two tier approach to biophysical assessment of the fetus. *Am J Obstet Gynecol* 1990;163:12–16.
26 van Geijn HP. Antepartum assessment of fetal condition by means of cardiotocography. *Curr Obstet Gynecol* 1997;7:87–92.
27 Aldrich CJ, Antona D, Spencer JAD *et al*. Late fetal heart decelerations and changes in cerebral oxygenation during the first stage of labour. *Br J Obstet Gynaecol* 1995;102:9–15.
28 Dawes GS, Moulden M, Redman CWG. The advantages of computerized fetal heart rate analysis. *J Perinat Med* 1991;19:39–45.
29 Dawes GS, Meir YJ, Mandruzzato GP. Computerized evaluation of fetal heart rate patterns. *J Perinat Med* 1994;22:491–9.
30 Alfrevic Z, Neilson JP. Doppler ultrasonography in high risk pregnancies: systematic review with meta-analysis. *Am J Obstet Gynecol* 1995;172: 1379–87.
31 Ramsay M. Use of Doppler ultrasound in antepartum assessment of the fetus. *Curr Obstet Gynecol* 1997;7:82–6.
32 Kingdom JCP, Rodeck CH, Kaufman P. Umbilical artery Doppler–more harm than good? *Br J Obstet Gynaecol* 1997;104:393–6.
33 Hecher K, Campbell S, Doyle P, Harrington K, Nicolaides K. Assessment of fetal compromise by Doppler ultrasound investigation of the fetal circulation. *Circulation* 1995;91:129–38.

4 Treatment of the Hypertensive Disorders of Pregnancy

D CHURCHILL AND DG BEEVERS

Introduction

There are still no clear guidelines stating when treatment for hypertension in pregnancy should be commenced, which are the best drugs to use as first and second line agents, for how long to continue with treatment and what levels of blood pressure should spark treatment in the non-acute situation. Despite the lack of clear guidance there is probably a fair degree of agreement when it comes to answering these questions. There will, however, be different areas of emphasis between clinicians depending upon which drugs and therapies individual clinicians have become accustomed to using.

In addition there are also a number of pitfalls and problems to avoid, or at least be aware of, when treating hypertensive pregnant women. No one drug is ideal. The number of randomised controlled trials carried out examining the treatment of hypertension in pregnancy is pitifully small. Therefore, one has to draw upon other types of evidence to guide one's choices for treatment. These include case control studies, prospective and retrospective follow-up studies, observational studies, and even case reports. Overall, in the majority of instances the choice of drug will be an easy one; however, it is useful before completing the prescription to consider whether the particular treatment chosen is appropriate for that individual.

The Principles of Treatment

Whenever there is more than one way of treating a specific condition, it is important for the doctor to be explicit and clear regarding the aims of treatment. Clearly the aims of treating severe hypertension in cases of fulminating pre-eclampsia are to prevent morbidity in and mortality of the mother and fetus.[1] In addition to this, the clinician treating the mother should also be specific about the levels of blood pressure which are clinically acceptable, the length of time for which treatment will be pursued, how the effect of the treatment will be monitored, and which criteria are to be used for adding in second line therapies or deciding upon delivery. The answers to these questions may be relatively easy in the case of fulminating pre-eclampsia. However, they are more difficult to answer when considering patients with mild to moderate pre-eclampsia or even chronic/essential hypertension diagnosed prior to 20 weeks' gestation. These questions become even more difficult to answer during the stages of a pregnancy when fetal viability is in the balance. In cases of pre-eclampsia the perceived risks from the disease to the mother must be weighed against those of prematurity for the fetus. Providing answers to these questions is extremely difficult and interventions can only be carried out after a great deal of thought.

Practice Point – Guiding Principles for Treatment of Hypertension in Pregnancy

- Decide on the unacceptable levels of blood pressure for each individual
- Fix the parameters of success, i.e. the blood pressure reduction required
- Fix the parameters of failure, i.e. for how long will drug treatment be pursued in the event of it failing to reduce blood pressure. This is especially important with pre-eclampsia prior to delivery
- Decide on how the effects of treatment will be monitored, outpatient or inpatient, and the frequency of measurements
- Decide the criteria for starting second line therapy

The guiding principle for most obstetricians is that the mother's life is of paramount importance. If this is to be put in jeopardy by prolonging a pregnancy, then fetal survival is a secondary consideration and terminating the pregnancy becomes the only viable option. Thankfully these situations only rarely occur and for the vast majority of mothers and babies the outcome is a happy one.

> **Practice Point – Aims of Treatment**
> - To prevent maternal morbidity and mortality
> - To prolong a pregnancy allowing fetal maturity to take place where this is safe; and thus to prevent and limit fetal morbidity and mortality

The Treatment of Essential/Chronic Hypertension

These patients can be divided into two groups, those who are known hypertensives prior to conception and will be referred early in pregnancy, probably on treatment, and those women in whom the hypertension is diagnosed during the first 20 weeks of pregnancy. The former group of patients should have already been investigated in an attempt to detect an underlying cause for its hypertension; the latter group needs to be investigated in order not to overlook any significant pathology. Generally it is usual not to alter the treatment a patient is already taking, unless the drug is positively dangerous to the fetus (or mother). This treatment may be continued until either changes are forced by a rise in blood pressure or there is the onset of acute superimposed pre-eclampsia.

The aim of treating chronic hypertension in pregnancy is to prevent accelerated placental atherosclerosis and thus prolong the pregnancy allowing greater fetal maturation. In addition it should protect the maternal cardiovascular system from the adverse effects of excessive fluctuations in blood pressure. An overview of the randomised controlled trials published in the Cochrane Database concluded that the treatment of chronic hypertension in pregnancy reduced the risk of development of severe hypertension (Figure 4.1). However, the trials were too small to comment upon the safety and efficacy of treatment using other more important outcome measures such as perinatal mortality.[2]

For women who develop chronic hypertension *de novo*, the decision upon which levels of blood pressure to treat is not absolute. A review of the database of hypertensive pregnancies over the past 18 years at the City Hospital, Birmingham has shown a greater tolerance of higher levels of diastolic pressure before

Comparisons and outcomes

Any antihypertensive therapy in chronic hypertension

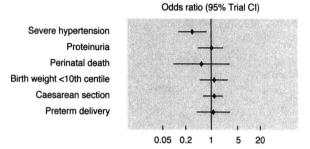

Figure 4.1 A meta-analysis of trials examining the treatment of chronic hypertension in pregnancy shows that the incidence of severe hypertension is reduced but overall there is no significant effect on perinatal mortality.

treatment is instituted. Our view is not to treat the hypertension unless the diastolic pressure is consistently over 95 mmHg to 100 mmHg. Close follow-up is, however, mandatory for all patients, whether they are being treated or not. Clearly there is a need for a randomised trial in order to determine the actual levels of pressure which need treating in these patients.

The Treatment of Pre-eclampsia

A more aggressive approach is taken to treating the hypertensive component of this condition. The aims are very clear: (a) to prevent maternal complications and (b) if safe, to prolong the pregnancy either to allow time for steroids to be administered or to allow natural maturation of the fetus to take place, thus preventing or attenuating the problem of respiratory distress syndrome in the neonate. This in turn further reduces the risks of the other complications from prematurity.[3] Once again the threshold of 95 mmHg of diastolic pressure triggers treatment, although we frequently treat lesser pressures in excess of 90 mmHg to achieve the stated aims. When treating pre-eclampsia, caution must be exercised. The pressure must not be lowered too far or too rapidly, as placental perfusion can be adversely affected and compromise the fetus. This is more likely to occur with intravenous therapy than with orally administered antihypertensives.

General Health of the Pregnant Hypertensive

While concentrating on treating the hypertension it is easy to forget that a pregnant woman can have other medical problems. These in turn can have effects that can lead to a rise in blood pressure. Therefore it is vital for the good management of these patients to ensure that they are generally as well as their condition allows.

Poor social circumstances, such as those commonly found with single parents or families with "no bread winner", cause a great deal of stress. Arranging help from the social service departments will often ease a troubled situation. This may then help with the management of the woman, by allowing her to attend for the necessary outpatient monitoring and improving compliance with prescribed treatments.

Anaemia in pregnancy is often a secondary phenomenon to a dilutional effect caused by the increase in plasma volume. However, iron deficiency is common and a haemoglobin below 11 g/dl is considered pathological. This leads to an increase in the pulse rate, and a further increase in cardiac output, which in turn results in an increase in blood pressure. This problem can be reduced or prevented by iron supplementation in those women who show the tendency towards anaemia.

The hypertensive group of women in particular should be encouraged to give up smoking. The detrimental effects upon the placenta and fetus may compound those which may be being caused by the ongoing placental pathology caused by hypertension.

Work can also be problematic. Nowadays it is an economic necessity in many families for the mother to work full time. Stopping work early has a disadvantageous effect on a woman's entitlement to maternity leave after the birth of the child. Both of these pressures force mothers to work longer into their pregnancies. Manual work in particular, where the mother is on her feet for many hours of the working day, has been shown to be detrimental and to lead to an increased tendency towards pre-eclampsia and future growth problems.[4] Women with hypertensive disorders in pregnancy should be encouraged to consider leaving work in the second trimester, allowing them to adopt a more sedentary and less stressful lifestyle in the later stages of their pregnancy. Alternatively help at home from the social services could have a beneficial effect.

Choice of Drug Treatment

Methyldopa

Dosages   *250 mg 2 to 3 times a day, gradually increasing as necessary over a period of 2 days to a maximum of 3 g per day*

Methyldopa is one of the oldest antihypertensive drugs and has an extensive track record in pregnancy. Nowadays it is used less frequently in the non-pregnant hypertensive woman. It acts on the brain stem as an alpha agonist to reduce sympathetic outflow activity. A randomised trial of methyldopa versus placebo for the treatment of moderate hypertension (defined as a BP of 150/95 mmHg) in pregnancy demonstrated an excess of perinatal deaths in the control group of patients.[5] The main effect was found in the group of individuals whose hypertension required treatment prior to 28 weeks' gestation. In the sub-group whose treatment was commenced after 28 weeks' gestation, the birth weight of the infants was higher in the treated group than the controls, as was the gestational age at delivery, but there were no differences in mortality. Overall, however, taking the group as a whole and adjusting for the duration of treatment, the birth and placental weights of the resulting infants were similar. The authors concluded that the treatment of moderate hypertension in pregnancy was safe with methyldopa and did confer some benefit on the treated individuals. The size of the study was small and as such prone to bias. Therefore the conclusions are still open to question, and other randomised trials using methyldopa have failed to show any benefit from treatment when compared to beta-blockers or no treatment.[6, 7]

Unlike most other antihypertensive drugs, the safety record of methyldopa in the long term has been investigated and shown to be sound.[8] One study followed up children of mothers who were treated during pregnancy with methyldopa, to the age of $7\frac{1}{2}$ years.[9] The outcome measures used in the study were the children's physical health, mental retardation, sight impairment, behavioural difficulties and the intelligence quotient. No significant differences were found between the children of treated mothers versus the children of control mothers.

Unfortunately, a major drawback with methyldopa is its side effect profile. Up to 22% of patients taking the drug suffer from depression, excessive sedation and/or postural hypotension. This causes problems with compliance and leads to 15% of patients discontinuing the treatment. In addition, a practical problem may be encountered when cross-matching a patient's blood, as methyldopa treatment causes a positive direct Coombes test. Cross-matching blood prior to treatment will overcome this annoying feature.

Beta-blockers

Labetalol   *dosage*   *400–800 mg daily in divided dosages*
Oxprenolol   *dosage*   *80–160 mg daily in divided dosages*

Beta-blockers are also widely used in pregnancy and in general terms are believed to be safe and effective.[10–12] They act upon both the heart and peripheral vasculature in order to lower blood pressure. Many clinicians have switched from methyldopa to this group of drugs because the side effects suffered are a less frequent occurrence. Randomised trials have confirmed their efficacy in controlling hypertension but in general they have been too small to show any distinct advantage over methyldopa as the first line treatment for hypertension during pregnancy.

Concerns have been raised over the effects beta-blockers may have on fetal haemodynamics. Those concerns have centred mainly on one of this group of drugs, atenolol. In a randomised controlled trial of atenolol versus pindolol the pulsatility index, a measure of resistance in the fetal circulation, was found to be raised in the umbilical artery and aorta of fetuses whose mothers were taking atenolol.[13] Also in this study the placental weights in the atenolol group were significantly reduced compared with the pindolol group. Further doubt was cast over the credentials of atenolol in a randomised placebo controlled trial for the treatment of chronic hypertension in pregnancy. The infant birth and placental weights of the atenolol arm were significantly reduced below those in the non-treatment arm.[14] Our own observational data have confirmed this finding.[15] The problem appears to be unique to atenolol, and when other beta-blockers have been studied, i.e. oxprenolol, pindolol and the alpha/beta-blocker labetalol, no such difficulties have been discovered.[16, 17] It has been postulated that atenolol has a specific inhibitory action on the placental growth factor human placental lactogen, although this has yet to be confirmed by experimental data. This adverse effect seems to be limited to those women who take atenolol in the long term, rather than in those who take it for a relatively short period of time during late pregnancy.

Because of the problems surrounding atenolol we have chosen labetalol as our first line beta-blocker for long term use in pregnancy. Its safety profile has not been questioned.[18] It has many of the actions of the non-selective beta-blockers and some alpha-adrenergic antagonist activity, which limits the broncho-constriction sometimes found with this group of drugs. Care still has to be taken when treating asthmatic patients, and in cases where the asthma is severe, it is better to choose an alternative to a beta-blocker in order to lower the blood pressure. In these instances methyldopa could be used.

Calcium channel antagonists

Nifedipine LA	*dosage*	*30–60 mg once daily*
Nifedipine	*dosage*	*10 mg 2–3 times a day*
Verapamil	*dosage*	*240–480 mg daily in divided doses*

Nifedipine is the most studied calcium channel blocker in pregnancy, although that is not to say others have not been used. We have personally managed patients taking verapamil and found no detrimental effects upon either the mother or fetus. Data from a retrospective study in 1987 found nifedipine to be an effective second line agent in controlling blood pressure after beta-blockers or methyldopa alone had failed.[19] Various trials have concluded that calcium channel blockers give better control of blood pressure in pregnancy than do the other available drugs. However, the methodology of these trials has been poor and it is difficult to be sure of their conclusions, particularly when comparing the drugs with those already studied much more extensively, like methyldopa and the beta-blockers. Nifedipine does appear to be safe and is consistently used as a second line agent in cases where the blood pressure is refractory to treatment and it is our opinion that it should continue to be used in this manner.

Nifedipine is also used in the acute situation of fulminating pre-eclampsia. While oral administration is acceptable, the sublingual form should not be used as absorption by the buccal or oesophageal mucosa is variable and unpredictable. Precipitate falls in blood pressure can occur causing a reduction in the blood flow through the uteroplacental circulation resulting in fetal distress. Even more worrying is that a large fall in the maternal blood pressure can compromise the maternal cerebral circulation, resulting in cerebrovascular accidents.

Thiazide diuretics

Diuretics have not been used for the treatment of hypertension in pregnancy for many years and there are good theoretical arguments against their use in PET. Pre-eclampsia is characterised by a depletion of the central intravascular volume. It is believed that diuretics could worsen this problem, causing deterioration in the patient's condition and further compromising the uteroplacental blood flow. In addition to this, the thiazide diuretics cause an elevation of the serum uric acid making it impossible to use the patient's serum level as an indicator of the severity of the disease.[20] On the other hand, a meta-analysis of the randomised controlled trials using these drugs has shown that there was no difference in the incidence of perinatal mortality or morbidity when compared with the controls (Figure 4.2).[21] The methodological quality of these trials was poor, but given the other disadvantages they are unlikely to be repeated in the foreseeable future.

Angiotensin converting enzyme inhibitors

This group of drugs is definitely contraindicated in pregnancy. There have been several reports of fetal and neonatal death as a result of renal failure and also teratogenesis in instances where angiotensin converting enzyme (ACE) inhibitors have been taken during conception. Skeletal dysplasias, particularly deficient skull ossification and limb reduction defects, seem to be drug specific abnormalities.[22] Data from the City hospital database, in which

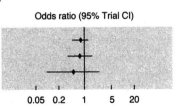

Figure 4.2 A meta-analysis of the treatment of pre-eclampsia with diuretics shows that no benefit is conferred in terms of mortality.

ACE inhibitors were taken in 18 pregnancies at the time of conception and during first trimester, revealed no excess skeletal deformities.[23] The risks of teratogenesis as determined from the case reports could have been affected by a degree of publication bias. From our own experience we would **not** encourage a woman to terminate a pregnancy on the basis of possible teratogenesis. ACE inhibitors should be stopped and the patient transferred to a suitable alternative antihypertensive drug when the pregnancy is confirmed. Where patients cannot be suitably reassured they can be offered prenatal diagnosis with ultrasound scanning, although this is not absolute, as some of the skeletal dysplasias cannot be identified by ultrasound until the later weeks of a pregnancy. Patients with pre-eclampsia may very well have compromised renal function with a reduction in glomerular filtration that could be aggravated by the ACE inhibitors.

Once the patient has been delivered, then ACE inhibitors may be used in the post partum period.

Practice Point – Treatment

General

- Social support for the single or poor etc.
- Ferrous sulphate supplements for anaemia
- Advice on when to stop work, tailored to the individual

Antihypertensives

- First line: methyldopa or a beta-blocker, e.g. labetalol or oxprenolol
- Second line: calcium channel blockers, e.g. nifedipine
- Avoid long term treatment with atenolol

In-patient Management and Delivery of Pre-eclamptic Women

Bed-rest has long been abandoned as a therapy for managing hypertensive pregnant women. However, many affected patients require hospitalisation for monitoring. If the patient is to co-operate fully with the wishes of her obstetrician and midwife, her confidence and morale needs to be maintained. This can only be achieved by keeping her fully informed about the disease process and sharing with her any areas of doubt or uncertainty regarding her management. Where possible, clear goals should be set, so that when the treatment is failing it can be appreciated by all involved. Any changes to the management plan will not then come as a complete surprise to the mother.

Hospitalised pre-eclamptic women are at increased risk of thromboembolic disease. Graduated TED stockings should be worn by these women and mobilisation encouraged. Those at very high risk, e.g. following a caesarean section, should have prophylactic subcutaneous heparin therapy in addition to stockings.

With careful maternal and fetal monitoring it should be possible to anticipate problems and allow the obstetrician enough time to plan a vaginal delivery. Ripening of the cervix with vaginal prostaglandin gel prior to a surgical induction is safe in most circumstances. During the labour both the maternal and fetal condition will need to be monitored assiduously. A significant deterioration in the condition of the mother, such as a rise in her blood pressure, needs treating promptly. If drug or fluid management fails to halt the deterioration in the maternal condition, then an operative delivery will become necessary.

In some cases where the blood pressure is successfully and readily controlled it may be possible to induce labour if the condition of the cervix is favourable. However, most antenatal patients with fulminating pre-eclampsia will need operative delivery, in order to prevent significant maternal and fetal morbidity or mortality. Before carrying out a caesarean section it is important to gain control over the blood pressure. Endotracheal intubation during general anaesthesia causes an acute rise in blood pressure, which needs to be limited to a minimum. A preferable alternative is regional anaesthesia via an epidural or spinal block, which will remove the problems associated with intubation and the risks of transplacental anaesthesia for the fetus. In addition, the intra-operative maternal blood loss tends to be reduced, as the generalised vasodilatory properties of the inhaled anaesthetics will obviously be avoided. Sometimes a caesarean section and its complications such as acute haemorrhage will complicate the management of patients with pre-eclampsia further. Coagulopathies may be worsened and fluid management made more difficult in these situations.

In pre-eclamptic patients undergoing a labour the fetal heart should be continuously monitored. The fetus may already be compromised and the added stress of uterine contractions may precipitate acute hypoxia. In these circumstances the fetus should be delivered immediately.

The Treatment of Acute Hypertensive Crises in Pregnancy

The most common form of hypertensive crisis in pregnancy is fulminating pre-eclampsia. This is a true obstetric emergency and these patients should be managed by a senior obstetrician, in collaboration with colleagues from the specialties of anaesthetics and medicine. These patients should be cared for where possible in a high dependency area on the labour ward. If there is not a suitable area on the labour ward then the main hospital high dependency unit (HDU) may be more appropriate. Each unit should have clearly laid down guidelines on how these patients should be managed. These guidelines should state the lines of responsibility, levels of blood pressure requiring treatment, drug regimens, fluid balance control, and methods of monitoring these patients. The majority of these cases will be of such a gestational age as to allow immediate delivery. This may very well be by caesarean section in the majority of cases and care of these women should also involve the appropriate postoperative management, to minimise the risk of thromboembolism and infection.

Whilst there is a paucity of evidence from randomised trials in this area, several workers have published their own experiences and observations. Details of the protocols we use are explained in the chapter dealing with intensive and high dependency care and only brief details will be outlined in this section.

For the treatment of hypertension we advocate the use of labetalol (100 mg orally three times a day or 50 mg intravenously) and hydralazine (5–10 mg intravenous boluses or an infusion titrated to the patient's blood pressure). We use labetalol in conjunction with hydralazine to limit the reactive tachycardia and systolic hypertension caused by the hydralazine. The hydralazine is given initially as boluses and only converted to an infusion when boluses fail to give adequate control.

The strongest evidence for the use of magnesium sulphate is for the prevention of recurrent fits in people with eclampsia. Based upon this evidence we believe that patients with severe PET, who exhibit more than one beat of clonus, will probably benefit from the administration of magnesium sulphate as a prophylactic agent against eclampsia. This view is contentious, as evidence for the use of the magnesium for severe pre-eclampsia is lacking. There is, however, light at the end of this particular tunnel. Currently under way is a randomised trial examining this question. The "MAGPIE" trial in which the authors' unit at Good Hope is a collaborating unit, aims to recruit several thousand pre-eclamptic women who will be randomised to receive either magnesium sulphate or placebo, to determine whether magnesium sulphate is safe and effective in the treatment of severe PET. The results of this particular trial will be valuable whatever the result and it is our view that it should be supported.[24]

Fluid management is as important as the treatment of hypertension in cases of fulminating PET. Again this will be discussed in greater detail in another chapter, but it is worth emphasising that the second highest cause of death from within this group of patients is adult respiratory distress syndrome (ARDS) as a result of iatrogenic fluid overload causing pulmonary oedema. Strict monitoring of fluid balance is mandatory in these patients.

Practice Point – Management of Acute Crises

- Senior clinicians should be involved directly in managing the patient
- Multi-specialty teams of obstetricians and anaesthetists are ideal, although others such as physicians may need to be called upon to help
- Patients should be managed in a HDU type area, preferably on the labour ward
- Each unit should have clear guidelines on the management of blood pressure, fluid balance, eclamptic convulsions, disseminated intravascular coagulopathies etc.
- Monitoring standards should include techniques and timings of: blood pressure measurement, fluid balance, oxygen saturation and the use of invasive monitoring such as arterial lines and central venous or Swan–Ganz catheterisation
- The guidelines should include prophylactic measures for preventing thrombosis, infection and gastric ulceration
- Where possible the management of these patients should be evidence based

---

Fetal and Neonatal Complications of Antihypertensive Treatment

Generally the antihypertensive agents have a good track record with regards to adverse effects upon the fetus and neonate. Methyldopa does cross the placenta and has been found in the amniotic fluid. No serious adverse effects have been reported and its long term safety has been proven.

Beta-blockers also cross the placenta, entering the fetal circulation and there have been anecdotal observations of neonatal morbidity, especially hypotension and hypoglycaemia. However these complications can also be due to prematurity alone. A thorough review by Rubin found that the anecdotal reports were unsubstantiated in prospective studies, which established the efficacy and safety of beta-blockers in pregnancy.[25] However, as previously stated, the long term use of atenolol has been associated with fetal growth retardation and therefore its use in pregnancy is best restricted to short term use only. This problem has not been noted with the other drugs in this group. Beta-blockers are also found in breast milk but in quantities that are clinically insignificant for the neonate and there is no reason to restrict breast-feeding.[26] Clinicians using the beta-blocking agents can take a fair degree of comfort from the evidence that these drugs are safe to take in pregnancy and the puerperium.

Practice Point – Drug Treatment

- Long term treatment with atenolol should be avoided due to its adverse effect on fetal and placental growth

---

Nifedipine has also been deemed to be safe for the fetus in pregnancy, though the body of evidence from which this conclusion is drawn is smaller than for the drugs previously mentioned. One potential problem which could become more significant in the future is its synergistic effect with magnesium sulphate. Therefore when they are given together, care must be exercised in order to prevent a precipitous fall in blood pressure. If this does occur, then fetal hypoxia could ensue from the concomitant fall in utero-placental perfusion.

Practice Point – Treatment

- Treatment with oral antihypertensive agents does not preclude a woman from breast-feeding her infant

---

Now that magnesium sulphate is increasingly being used in the UK, the effects upon the fetus and neonate are becoming of interest. Serum magnesium levels in the fetus equilibrate with the levels found in the mother and have the potential to cause respiratory depression. This has been shown to be an unlikely consequence of therapy with magnesium, although continuous intravenous infusions in the mother do cause neonatal hypermagnesaemia.[27, 28] The clearance of the magnesium from the infant's circulation is prolonged, but at normal doses does not cause a deleterious effect upon the newborn.[29]

Summary

General health care is just as important when managing pregnant women, as is treating any hypertension. From the published evidence we feel that it is impossible to favour either methyldopa or a beta-blocker as the first line antihypertensive agent in pregnancy. We choose a beta-blocker over methyldopa because of the latter's problematic side effect profile and reduced compliance. Labetalol or oxprenolol give good control and when used in conjunction with hydralazine in the acute situation prevent the reactive systolic hypertension. Having said that, if there is a contraindication to the use of beta-blockers, e.g. maternal asthma, then methyldopa would be our alternative first line agent. We generally avoid atenolol because of its adverse effects on fetal growth when used in the long term. The second line agent of choice, should either labetalol or methyldopa fail to control the blood pressure adequately, is nifedipine.

Before treating any woman, however, the clinician must be clear about what exactly he or she is hoping to achieve and be ready to deliver the fetus if treatment is seen to be failing. Nothing is to be gained from lowering the blood pressure in a pre-eclamptic patient if the other effects of the disease process on the body's other systems are running out of control.

References

1 *Report on Confidential Enquiries into Maternal Deaths in the United Kingdom 1991–1993*. London: HMSO, 1996.
2 Duley L. Any antihypertensive therapy in chronic hypertension (revised 2 June 1992). In: Keirse MJNC, Renfrew MJ, Neilson JP, Crowther C, eds. *Pregnancy and childbirth module. The Cochrane pregnancy and childbirth database*. The Cochrane Collaboration Issue 2. Oxford: Update Software, 1995. (Available from BMJ Publishing Group, London.)

3 Crowley P. Corticosteroids prior to preterm delivery (revised 19 August 1994). In: Keirse MJNC, Renfrew MJ, Neilson JP, Crowther C, eds. *Pregnancy and childbirth module. The Cochrane pregnancy and childbirth database.* The Cochrane Collaboration Issue 2. Oxford: Update Software, 1995. (Available from BMJ Publishing Group, London.)

4 Klonoff-Cohen HS, Cross JL, Pieper CF. Job stress and pre-eclampsia. *Epidemiology* 1996;7:245–9.

5 Redman CWG, Beilin LJ, Bonnar J, Ounsted MK. Fetal outcome in trial of antihypertensive treatment in pregnancy. *Lancet* 1976;ii:753–6.

6 Sibai BM, Mabie WC, Shamsa F, Villar MA, Anderson GD. A comparison of no medication versus methyldopa or labetolol in chronic hypertension during pregnancy. *Am J Obstet Gynecol* 1990;162:960–7.

7 Gallery EDM, Saunders DM, Hunyor SN, Gyorgy AZ. Randomised comparison of methyldopa and oxprenolol for the treatment of hypertension in pregnancy. *Br Med J* 1979;i:1591–4.

8 Cockburn J, Moar VA, Ounsted M, Redman CWG. Final report of study on hypertension during pregnancy: the effects of specific treatment on growth and development of the children. *Lancet* 1982;i:647–9.

9 Ounsted M, Cockburn J, Moar VA, Redman CWG. Maternal hypertension with superimposed pre-eclampsia: effects on child development at $7\frac{1}{2}$ years. *Br J Obstet Gynaecol* 1983;90:644–9.

10 Tcherdakoff PH, Colliard M, Berrard E, Kreft C, Dupay A, Bernaille JM. Propranolol in hypertension during pregnancy. *Br Med J* 1978;ii:670.

11 Rubin PC. Current concepts: beta-blockers in pregnancy. *N Engl J Med* 1981;305:1323–6.

12 Pickles CJ, Symonds EM, Broughton-Pipkin F. The fetal outcome in a randomized double-blind controlled trial of labetalol versus placebo in pregnancy induced hypertension. *Br J Obstet Gynaecol* 1989;96:38–43.

13 Montan S, Ingemarsson I, Marsal K, Sjoberg NO. Randomised controlled trial of atenolol and pindolol in human pregnancy: effects on fetal haemodynamics. *Br Med J* 1992;304:946–9.

14 Rubin PC, Butters L, Clark DM *et al.* Placebo controlled trial of atenolol in treatment of pregnancy associated hypertension. *Lancet* 1983;i:431.

15 Lip GHY, Beevers M, Churchill D, Shaffer L, Beevers DG. Effect of atenolol on birth weight. *Am J Cardiol* 1997;79:47–9.

16 Jouppila P, Kirkinen P, Koivula A, Ylikorkala O. Labetalol does not alter placental and fetal blood flow or maternal prostanoids in pre-eclampsia. *Br J Obstet Gynaecol* 1986;93:543–7.

17 Plouin PF, Breart G, Llado J *et al.* A randomized comparison of early with conservative use of anti-hypertensive drugs in the management of pregnancy induced hypertension. *Br J Obstet Gynaecol* 1990;97:134–41.

18 MacPherson M, Broughton-Pipkin F, Rutter N. The effect of maternal labetalol on the newborn infant. *Br J Obstet Gynaecol* 1986;93:539–42.

19 Constantine G, Beevers DG, Reynolds AC. Nifedipine as a second line antihypertensive drug in pregnancy. *Br J Obstet Gynaecol* 1987;94:1136–42.

20 Rubin PC. Treatment of hypertension in pregnancy. *Clin Obstet Gynaecol* 1986;13:307–17.

21 Duley L. Diuretics in the treatment of pre-eclampsia (revised 29 April 1993). In: Keirse MJNC, Renfrew MJ, Neilson JP, Crowther C, eds. *Pregnancy and childbirth module. The Cochrane pregnancy and childbirth database.* The Cochrane Collaboration Issue 2. Oxford: Update Software, 1995. (Available from BMJ Publishing Group, London.)

22 Hanssens M, Keirse MJNC, Vankelecom F, van Assche FA. Fetal and neonatal effects of treatment with angiotensin converting enzyme inhibitors in pregnancy. *Obstet Gynecol* 1991;78:128.

23 Lip GYH, Churchill D, Beevers M, Auckett A, Beevers DG. Angiotensin-converting enzyme inhibitors in early pregnancy. *Lancet* 1997;**350**:1446–7.

24 Duley L. The MAGPIE trial: magnesium sulphate versus placebo for women with pre-eclampsia. *Br J Obstet Gynaecol* 1998;**105** (Suppl 17):40.

25 Rubin PC. Beta-blockers in pregnancy. *N Engl J Med* 1981;**305**:1323.

26 White BW, Andreoli JW, Wong SH, Cohn RD. Atenolol in human plasma and breast milk. *Obstet Gynecol* 1984;**63**:425.

27 Stone SR, Pritchard JA. Effect of maternally administered magnesium sulphate on the neonate. *Obstet Gynecol* 1970;**35**:574.

28 Lipsitz PJ. The clinical and biochemical effects of excess magnesium in the newborn. *Paediatrics* 1977;**47**:501.

29 Dangman BC, Rosen TS. Magnesium levels in infants of mothers treated with magnesium sulphate. *Pediatr Res* 1977;**11**:415.

5　Pathogenesis of Pre-eclampsia

K BRACKLEY AND MD KILBY

Introduction

Pre-eclampsia, a systemic disorder associated with pregnancy, is characterised by the development of hypertension and proteinuria after 20 weeks' gestation, with reversal of this disease state to normal in the puerperium. This disease is a major cause of maternal morbidity and mortality and is associated with increased perinatal problems because of intrauterine growth restriction and preterm delivery. Despite a wealth of research the exact cause of pre-eclampsia remains unknown and it has been aptly referred to as the "disease of theories".[1]

This chapter will review a variety of theories concerning the pathogenesis of pre-eclampsia with particular emphasis on more recent developments.

Genetic Predisposition

Although the genetic basis of this disorder is unclear, epidemiological studies suggest that the disease predominates in first pregnancies of women who are homozygous for a "susceptibility gene".[2] Although there has been evidence that women of blood group AB are significantly more susceptible to pre-eclampsia,[3] HLA-G deletion polymorphism investigations of pedigrees have noted no detectable susceptibility.[4]

Angiotensinogen exhibits genetic linkage to and association with essential hypertension. In pre-eclamptic patients, a mutation causing a molecular variant of angiotensinogen, T235, was identified.[5] However, subsequent review in a cohort of high-risk subjects who had a positive second trimester angiotensin II pressor test showed no such significant association.[6] The search for a candidate gene or gene-deletion continues.

Impaired Implantation

Between 12 and 20 weeks' gestation in "normal" pregnancy there is invasion of the maternal spiral uterine arteries by extravillous cytotrophoblasts as far as the myometrial segments. This process converts the narrow-diameter spiral arteries into distended unresponsive uteroplacental vessels, able to accommodate the vast increase in uterine blood flow requirements during pregnancy (Figure 5.1). There is histological evidence that in women who later develop pre-eclampsia there has been defective penetration by the cytotrophoblast so that these maternally derived arteries retain the musculoelastic elements of their walls (Figure 5.2)[7, 8] In placental bed biopsies from pre-eclamptic pregnancies in the third trimester, the endothelial lining of these arteries appears to be focally disrupted by attached intraluminal endovascular

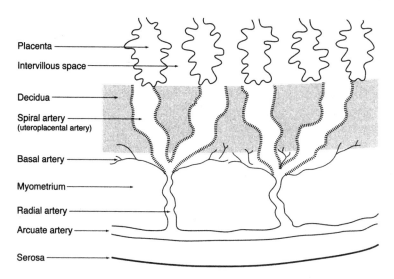

Figure 5.1   Diagram of the blood supply to the placenta in the third trimester. The spinal arteries (hatched) have been converted to uteroplacental arteries from their origins from the radial arteries. (Reproduced with permission from Gerretsen G, Huisjes HJ, Elema JD. Morphological changes of the spiral arteries in the placental bed in relation to pre-eclampsia and fetal growth retardation. *Br J Obstet Gynaecol* 1981; **88**:876–81.)

trophoblast.[9] However, it should be noted that endovascular trophoblast invasion is not an "all or none" phenomenon in normal and pre-eclamptic pregnancies and that probably a spectrum of invasion and spiral artery morphological change occurs.[10]

The cause of this impaired "placentation" is not fully understood but may be due to poor invasive properties of the trophoblastic cells or changes in the maternal decidual tissues which regulate trophoblast behaviour, perhaps mediated via multifunctional cytokine pathways (see growth factors). The cytotrophoblastic expression of adhesion molecules which influence invasion is altered in women with pre-eclampsia.[11] *In vitro* studies have shown lower attachment of trophoblasts from pre-eclamptic placentas on fibronectin and vitronectin compared to normotensive controls, which may reflect differences in expression of matrix receptors.[12] Maternal factors leading to inhibition of trophoblast invasion include reduced expression of the histocompatibility antigen

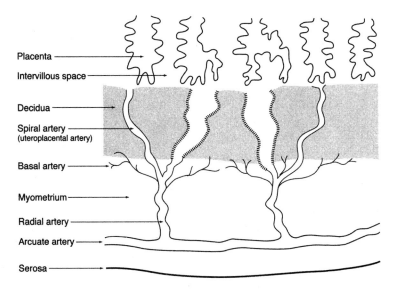

Figure 5.2   Diagram of the blood supply to the placenta in pre-eclampsia: the spiral arteries are either not converted to uteroplacental arteries (solid outlines) or, if they are, have been so converted only in their decidual segments (hatched outlines). (Reproduced with permission from Gerretson G, Huisjes HJ, Elema JD. Morphological changes of the spiral arteries in the placental bed in relation to pre-eclampsia and fetal growth retardation. *Br J Obstet Gynaecol* 1981; **88**:876–81.)

HLA-G,[13] local inflammatory cell behaviour[14, 15] and cytokine regulation of integrin expression.[16]

Endothelial disruption within the placenta will predispose to platelet aggregation, vasospasm and thrombosis. The balance between endothelial release of vasoconstrictors such as endothelin and thromboxane and vasodilators such as prostacyclin and nitric oxide are altered in pre-eclampsia in favour of vasoconstriction[17] (see below). The combined effects of the above changes are a reduction in uteroplacental perfusion and possibly a relatively hypoxic placenta, particularly in later pregnancy. Maternal vascular diseases, such as autoimmune disorders and chronic hypertension, and multiple pregnancy with an increased trophoblastic tissue mass all predispose to pre-eclampsia, possibly due to a comparable reduction in uteroplacental blood flow.

These ischaemic conditions could be linked to the release of some factor(s) from the placenta into the maternal circulation. This factor subsequently causes, directly or indirectly, widespread endothelial damage and dysfunction which are the hallmarks of the maternal manifestations of pre-eclampsia.

Growth Factors

Growth factors are substances which have effects at a cellular level, many of which are by autocrine or paracrine mechanisms. Vascular endothelial growth factor (VEGF) is a potent angiogenic cytokine, inducing endothelial cell proliferation and chemotaxis, as well as vasculo- and angiogenesis.[18] The mRNA encoding VEGF[19] and protein[20] are expressed by human villous and extravillous trophoblast, while mRNA encoding the receptor (flt-1) is highly expressed in the cytotrophoblast shell and columns and also in some trophoblast cell lines (BeWo).[21] It has been suggested that trophoblast expresses high mRNA levels of VEGF and this causes endothelial cells which express flt-1 to migrate towards it. In third trimester placental biopsies the expression of VEGF mRNA has been demonstrated to be reduced in pre-eclamptic pregnancies and a significant negative correlation exists with increasing gestation. In contrast, trophoblast flt-1 mRNA expression was unaltered in pre-eclampsia.[22] It may be that VEGF is at least in part responsible for the deficient development of the terminal villi and reduced capillary branching in placentae of pre-eclamptic pregnancies. It may be that other non-heparin bound "angiogenic" growth factors also play a role in trophoblastic development and migration in trophoblast–vascular interaction in pre-eclamptic pregnancies[23].

Endothelial Dysfunction

Evidence of altered endothelial cell function in pre-eclampsia includes activation of the coagulation cascade, increased membrane permeability, enhanced response to pressor agents and increased vasoconstriction, which all contribute to reduced perfusion of affected organs including kidney, liver, and brain.[24, 25] Increased levels of substances known to be released from activated or injured endothelial cells have been described in pre-eclampsia, supporting this concept. These markers of endothelial damage include fibronectin,[26–30] laminin,[26] tissue plasminogen activator, plasminogen activator inhibitor-1[30] and von Willebrand factor.[28, 30] Indeed certain markers of endothelial damage and platelet activation are increased some weeks before the onset of clinical symptoms.[26]

There is an increased turnover of platelets in normal pregnancy which is accelerated in pre-eclampsia together with enhanced activation of the coagulation cascade.[31] Damaged endothelial surfaces will encourage platelet adherence and clot formation. Platelet activation will give rise to more mitogens, such as platelet-derived growth factors, vasoconstricting agents such as thromboxane and serotonin, and procoagulants, thus accelerating the process. The resulting vasospasm and microthrombi will cause additional endothelial cell damage which will further reduce uteroplacental blood flow, giving rise to a vicious circle of events.

There is an increased production of vasoconstrictors and a reduced synthesis of vasodilators in pre-eclampsia which, together with the enhanced response to vasopressor agents,[32, 33] results in a marked increase in vascular smooth muscle tone. Circulating levels of endothelin, a potent vasoconstrictor produced by endothelial cells, are higher in pre-eclampsia.[34–36] The levels are correlated to markers of disease severity, including plasma urate, serum creatinine and creatinine clearance levels.[37] The ratio between thromboxane, a vasoconstrictor and powerful platelet aggregating agent, and prostacyclin, a potent vasodilator and inhibitor of platelet aggregation, is increased in pre-eclampsia both in the maternal circulation and in the placenta.[17, 27, 38–40] This imbalance has been linked to the greater sensitivity of the vasculature to angiotensin II.[41]

Nitric Oxide and Pre-eclampsia

The role of nitric oxide in the pathogenesis of pre-eclampsia has been comprehensively reviewed.[42] Nitric oxide is a powerful vasodilator released by the endometrium and is believed to contribute to the generalised vasodilatation seen in normal pregnancy. The isoform of nitric oxide synthase released from the endothelium (eNOS) is constitutive (always present) and calcium-dependent. Nitric oxide generated in the endothelium causes vasodilatation and reduces the affinity of the endothelium to platelets. Activated platelets will increase eNOS activity and thereby control platelet aggregation and adherence to the endothelium. Evidence for an altered nitric oxide production in pregnancy originated in animal studies. Calcium-dependent NOS activity rises in animal pregnancy.[43] Conrad et al.[44] reported increased plasma levels and urinary excretion of cGMP as well as increased nitric oxide synthesis in pregnant rats. In human pregnancy NOS activity has been demonstrated in the placenta[45-48] and in the endothelium of the umbilical vessels.[48]

Chronic blockade of nitric oxide synthesis in pregnant rats produces a syndrome similar to pre-eclampsia with sustained hypertension, proteinuria, thrombocytopenia, decreased plasma volume, increased sensitivity to pressor agents, and evidence of placental insufficiency.[49-52]

Conflicting results have arisen in the literature concerning the changes in nitric oxide synthesis in hypertensive pregnancies. For example, lower plasma nitrite levels have been found in pre-eclampsia by some authors[53] but others have found no changes compared to normotensive pregnancy.[54] Cameron et al.[55] detected no significant differences in the urinary excretion of nitric oxide metabolites between hypertensive and normotensive pregnant women. However, a positive correlation was noted between urinary nitrate and nitrite excretion and change in systolic blood pressure, suggesting a compensatory increase in nitric oxide synthesis in hypertension. In a more recent study, in which concomitant measurement of plasma and urinary nitric oxide metabolites was performed as well as adjustment for differences in renal function between patients, urinary excretion of nitrites and nitrates was reduced in pre-eclampsia compared to normal pregnancy.[56] No differences were found in plasma nitric oxide metabolites between subject groups, implying a decrease in nitric oxide production in pre-eclampsia. Some of these discrepancies may have arisen because of different methodologies and lack of conformity between patient groups in terms of diet and disease categorisation.

A reduction in NOS activity within the placenta[57] has been described in pre-eclampsia. Impaired release of nitric oxide from perfused umbilical vessels occurred in response to bradykinin.[58] However although total calcium-dependent nitric oxide production by umbilical vein endothelial cells was lower in pre-eclampsia, the maximum nitric oxide production capacity of individual endothelial cells was apparently unaffected.[59] Indeed, a significant increase in serum nitrite concentration has been reported in umbilical venous serum in pre-eclampsia compared to normal pregnancy.[54] It was proposed that an increase in nitric oxide production in the fetoplacental circulation may be a compensatory mechanism to increase blood flow or to help modify platelet adhesion and aggregation in the disease.

What is "Factor X"?

A variety of *in vitro* experiments support the concept of a circulating factor in the blood of pre-eclamptic women which gives rise to the generalised endothelial cell dysfunction.[25] Sera from pre-eclamptic women induce changes in certain metabolic and functional properties of cultured endothelial cells, including increased release of fibronectin,[60, 61] increased intracellular triglyceride concentrations and the stimulation of platelet-derived growth factor mRNA and protein production.[60, 62] Paradoxically, the production of prostacyclin by cultured endothelial cells, both umbilical vein and decidual, is enhanced by initial incubation over 24 hours with pre-eclamptic sera or plasma.[63–65] However, longer exposure over 72 hours resulted in inhibition of endothelial prostacyclin production.[66] Increased nitrite production associated with elevated expression of endothelial NO synthase (eNOS) has been observed in cultured endothelial cells exposed to plasma from women with pre-eclampsia compared to plasma from normal pregnant women.[67, 68] However, the dangers in extrapolating these findings to the *in vivo* situation was highlighted by a recent series of experiments reported by Baker *et al.*[69] The application of shear stress increased both prostacyclin and nitric oxide production by endothelial cells, resulting in no significant differences detected when comparing exposure to plasma from normal pregnant or pre-eclamptic subjects.

The nature of the putative factor in the maternal circulation causing the extensive endothelial damage has not been determined. Proposed agents include syncytiotrophoblast microvillous membranes shed into the maternal blood perfusing the placenta.[70] Trophoblasts have been demonstrated in the maternal circulation with increased amounts in the uterine vein in pre-eclampsia compared to normal pregnancy.[71] Certainly the surface of the placenta in pre-eclampsia has abnormally shaped microvilli with focal areas of necrosis[72] and it has been demonstrated that preparations of these membranes inhibit endothelial cell growth *in vitro* analogous to the effect of plasma from pre-eclamptic women.[70, 73]

The activation of neutrophils in the decidua may release substances into the maternal blood which cause the endothelial damage in pre-eclampsia. These substances could include toxic proteases such as elastase from neutrophil granules,[15, 74] cell adhesion molecules such as VCAM-1,[75, 76] or cytokines such as interleukin-1, interleukin-6[75] and tissue necrosis factor-α.[77]

The levels of circulating lipid peroxides are higher in pre-eclampsia compared to normal pregnancy and are an alternative mechanism for producing the endothelial dysfunction.[78] The placental production of lipid peroxides by trophoblastic cells is increased in pre-eclampsia and presumably greater amounts are secreted into the maternal blood.[40] In addition, lipid peroxides can activate neutrophils as they circulate through the intervillous space leading to the release of superoxide anions which also cause membrane lipid peroxidation.[74, 79]

Lipid Peroxidation and Fatty Acid Metabolism in Pre-eclampsia

In normal pregnancy there is an increase in triglyceride synthesis in the liver following an increased flux of free fatty acids and reduced fatty acid oxidation. A compensatory secretion of very low density lipoprotein (VLDL) occurs which is further enhanced in pre-eclampsia, when higher levels of free fatty acids and triglycerides are found,[80] even weeks before the disease is clinically detectable.[81] A higher level of free fatty acids to albumin has been demonstrated in the sera of women with pre-eclampsia as well as increased lipolytic activity.[82] These factors resulted in greater triglyceride accumulation in cultured endothelial cells. Triglyceride accumulation alters endothelial cell function *in vitro* as shown by a reduction in prostacyclin release.[83] More specifically, linoleic acid, one of the circulating free fatty acids which is increased in pre-eclampsia, has been shown to impair basal cyclic guanylate monophosphate production and inhibit platelet aggregation, as well as reduce prostacyclin release.[84]

The balance between lipid peroxidation and protective anti-oxidant activity is changed in pre-eclampsia compared to normal pregnancy. An increase in lipid peroxides occurs in pre-eclampsia[85] together with a decrease in antioxidant activity.[39, 86, 87] The greater degree of lipid peroxidation probably reflects the higher levels of circulating lipids in this condition.[80]

Lipid peroxides are very unstable toxic compounds and can affect endothelial cell function by various mechanisms which are all associated with pre-eclampsia. Lipid peroxides and oxygen-free radicals can alter cell membrane fluidity and permeability[88] and promote platelet aggregation. Both prostacyclin synthase and cyclo-oxygenase enzymes are inhibited by elevated levels of lipid peroxides with a subsequent reduction in endothelial prostacyclin release, contributing to the altered thromboxane/prostacyclin ratio in pre-eclampsia.[39] Lipid peroxides can increase the passage of calcium onto cells and potentiate vasoconstriction.[89]

In addition to the increased concentration of VLDL in the circulation in pre-eclampsia, levels of small dense LDL are higher, this is particularly susceptible to oxidation. Both VLDL and LDL are known to cause endothelial damage and have therefore been suggested as causative agents in the disease (see Sattar *et al.* for recent review[90]). Oxidised LDL enhances adherence of neutrophils to endothelium and induces interleukin-1b release from mono-nuclear cells. It can also inhibit prostacyclin synthesis, increase endothelin production and inactivate nitric oxide. Oxidised VLDL increases synthesis of PAI-1 and together with LDL gives rise to platelet activation.

Summary

The primary event in the development of pre-eclampsia appears to be an abnormal trophoblastic invasion early on in pregnancy. The underlying causes of this defective implantation have not been clearly defined but are believed to result in hypoxic conditions within the placenta which subsequently lead to the release of an unknown factor(s) into the maternal circulation. The nature of this factor remains elusive but it is thought to be the agent giving rise to the generalised endothelial dysfunction which is strongly associated with pre-eclampsia. The roles of altered nitric oxide production and abnormal lipoprotein metabolism in the pathophysiology of the disease demand further study. It is only by understanding the processes underlying this important disease in pregnancy that it will ever be possible to predict and, more importantly, prevent pre-eclampsia.

References

1 Broughton-Pipkin F, Rubin PC. Pre-eclampsia – the "disease of theories". *Br Med Bull* 1994;**50**:381–96.

2 Hayward C, Livingstone J, Holloway S, Liston WA, Brock DJH. An exclusion map for pre-eclampsia: assuming autosomal recessive inheritance. *Am J Hum Genet* 1992;**50**:749–57.

3 Spinillo A, Capuzzo E, Baltaro F, Piazzi G, Iasci A. A case-control study of maternal blood group and severe pre-eclampsia. *J Hum Hypertens* 1995;**9**:623–5.

4 Humphreys KE, Harrison GA, Cooper DW et al. HLA-G deletion polymorphism and pre-eclampsia. *Br J Obstet Gynaecol* 1995;**102**:707–10.

5 Ward K, Hata A, Jeunemaitre X et al. A molecular variant of angiotensinogen associated with pre-eclampsia. *Nature Genetics* 1993;**4**:59–61.

6 Morgan L, Baker PN, Broughton-Pipkin F, Kalsheker N. Pre-eclampsia and the angiotensinogen gene. *Br J Obstet Gynaecol* 1995;**102**:489–90.

7 Brosens IA. Morphological changes in the utero-placental bed in pregnancy hypertension. *Clin Obstet Gynaecol* 1977;**4**:573–93.

8 Redman CWG. Current topic: pre-eclampsia and the placenta. *Placenta* 1991;**12**:301–8.

9 Khong TY, Sawyer IH, Heryet AR. An immunohistologic study of endothelialization of uteroplacental vessels in human pregnancy – evidence that endothelium is focally disrupted by trophoblast in pre-eclampsia. *Am J Obstet Gynecol* 1992;**167**:751–6.

10 Meekins JW, Pijnenborg R, Hanssens M, McFadyen IR, van Assche FA. A study of placental bed spiral arteries and trophoblast invasion in normal and severe pre-eclamptic pregnancies. *Br J Obstet Gynaecol* 1994;**101**:669–74.

11 Zhou Y, Damsky CH, Chiu K, Roberts JM, Fisher SJ. Pre-eclampsia is associated with abnormal expression of adhesion molecules by invasive cytotrophoblasts. *J Clin Invest* 1993;**91**:950–60.

12 Pijnenborg R, Luyten C, Vercruysse L, Van Assche FA. Attachment and differentiation *in vitro* of trophoblast from normal and pre-eclamptic human placentas. *Am J Obstet Gynecol* 1996;**175**:30–6.

13 Colbern GT, Chiang MH, Main EK. Expression of the nonclassic histocompatibility antigen HLA-G by pre-eclamptic placenta. *Am J Obstet Gynecol* 1994;**170**:1244–50.

14 Johnston TA, Greer IA, Dawes J, Calder AA. Neutrophil activation in small for gestational age pregnancies. *Br J Obstet Gynaecol* 1991;**98**:104–5.

15 Butterworth BH, Greer IA, Liston WA, Haddad NG, Johnston TA. Immunocytochemical localization of neutrophil elastase in term placenta, decidua, and myometrium in pregnancy induced hypertension. *Br J Obstet Gynaecol* 1991;**98**:929–33.

16 Vinatier D, Monnier JC. Pre-eclampsia: physiology and immunological aspects. *Eur J Obstet Gynecol Reprod Biol* 1995;**61**:85–97.

17 Walsh SW. Pre-eclampsia: an imbalance in placental prostacyclin and thromboxane production. *Am J Obstet Gynecol* 1985;**152**:335–40.

18 Ferrara N, Houck K, Jakeman L, Leung DW. The molecular and biological properties of VEGF family of proteins. *Endocrinol Rev* 1992;**13**:18–32.

19 Sharkey AM, Charnock-Jones DS, Boocock CA, Brown KD, Smith SK. Expression of VEGF in human placenta. *J Reprod Fertil* 1993;**99**:609–15.

20 Ahmed AS, Li X-F, Dunk C, Whittle MJ, Rushton DI, Rollason T. Colocalisation of VEGF and its flt-1 receptor in the human placenta. *Growth Factors* 1995;**12**:235–43.

21 Charnock-Jones DS, Sharkey AM, Boocock CA, Smith SK. VEGF receptor localisation and activation in human trophoblast and choriocarcinoma cell lines. *Biol Reprod* 1994;**51**:524–30.

22 Cooper JC, Sharkey AM, Charnock-Jones DS, Palmer CR, Smith SK. VEGF mRNA levels in placentae from pregnancies complicated by pre-eclampsia. *Br J Obstet Gynaecol* 1996;**103**:1191–6.

23 Ahmed A, Kilby MD. Hypoxia or hyperoxia in placental insufficiency. *Lancet* 1997; **350**:826–7.

24 Roberts JM, Taylor RN, Musci TJ, Rodgers GM, Hubel CA, McLaughlin MK. Pre-eclampsia: an endothelial cell disorder. *Am J Obstet Gynecol* 1989;**161**:1200–4.

25 Roberts JM, Redman CWG. Pre-eclampsia: more than pregnancy-induced hypertension. *Lancet* 1993;**341**:1447–51.

26 Ballegeer VC, Spitz B, de Baene LA, van Assche FA, Hidajat M, Criel AM. Platelet activation and vascular damage in gestational hypertension. *Am J Obstet Gynecol* 1992;**166**:629–33.

27 Kraayenbrink AA, Dekker GA, van Kamp GJ, van Geijn HP. Endothelial vasoactive mediators in preeclampsia. *Am J Obstet Gynecol* 1993;**169**:160–5.

28 Deng L, Bremme K, Hansson LO, Blomback M. Plasma levels of von Willebrand factor and fibronectin as markers of persisting endothelial damage in preeclampsia. *Obstet Gynecol* 1994;**84**:941–5.

29 Friedman SA, de Groot CJM, Taylor RN, Golditch BD, Roberts JM. Plasma cellular fibronectin as a measure of endothelial involvement in pre-eclampsia and intrauterine growth retardation. *Am J Obstet Gynecol* 1994;**170**:838–41.

30 Friedman SA, Schiff E, Emeis JJ, Dekker GA, Sibai BM. Biochemical corroboration of endothelial involvement in severe pre-eclampsia. *Am J Obstet Gynecol* 1995;**172**:202–3.

31 Redman CWG, Denson KWE, Beilin LJ, Bolton FG, Stirrat GM. Factor-VIII consumption in pre-eclampsia. *Lancet* 1977;**ii**:1249–52.

32 Gant NF, Daley GL, Chand S, Whalley PJ, MacDonald PC. A study of angiotensin II pressor response throughout primigravid pregnancy. *J Clin Invest* 1973;**52**:2682–9.

33 Worley RJ, Gant NF, Everett RB, MacDonald PC. Vascular responsiveness to pressor agents during human pregnancy. *J Reprod Med* 1979;**23**:115–28.

34 Nova A, Sibai BM, Barton JR, Mercer BM, Mitchell MD. Maternal plasma level of endothelin is increased in preeclampsia. *Am J Obstet Gynecol* 1991;**165**:724–7.

35 Mastrogiannis DS, O'Brien WF, Krammer J, Benoit R. Potential role of endothelin–1 in normal and hypertensive pregnancies. *Am J Obstet Gynecol* 1991;**165**:1711–16.

36 Schiff E, Ben-Baruch G, Peleg E *et al.* Immunoreactive circulating endothelin–1 in normal and hypertensive pregnancies. *Am J Obstet Gynecol* 1992;**166**:624–8.

37 Clark BA, Halvorson L, Sachs B, Epstein FH. Plasma endothelin levels in pre-eclampsia: elevation and correlation with uric acid levels and renal impairment. *Am J Obstet Gynecol* 1992;**166**:962–8.

38 Fitzgerald DJ, Entman SS, Mulloy K. Decreased prostacyclin biosynthesis preceding the clinical manifestation of pregnancy-induced hypertension. *Circulation* 1987;**75**:956–63.

39 Wang Y, Walsh SW, Guo J, Zhang J. The imbalance between thromboxane and

prostacyclin in pre-eclampsia is associated with an imbalance between lipid peroxides and vitamin E in maternal blood. *Am J Obstet Gynecol* 1991;**165**:1695–700.

40 Walsh SW, Wang Y. Trophoblast and placental villous core production of lipid peroxides, thromboxane and prostacyclin in preeclampsia. *J Clin Endocrinol Metabol* 1995;**80**:1888–93.

41 Everett RB, Worley RJ, MacDonald PC, Gant NF. Effect of prostaglandin synthetase inhibitors on pressor response to angiotensin II in human pregnancy. *J Clin Endocrinol Metabol* 1978;**46**:1007–10.

42 Morris NH, Eaton BM, Dekker G. Nitric oxide, the endothelium, pregnancy and pre-eclampsia. *Br J Obstet Gynaecol* 1996;**103**:4–15.

43 Weiner CP, Lizasoain I, Baylis SA, Knowles RG, Charles IG, Moncada S. Induction of calcium-dependent nitric oxide synthases by sex hormones. *Proc Natl Acad Sci USA* 1994;**91**:5212–16.

44 Conrad KP, Vernier KA. Plasma level, urinary excretion and metabolic production of cGMP during gestation in rats. *Am J Physiol* 1989;**257**:R847-53.

45 Conrad KP, Vill M, McGuire PG, Dail WG, Davis AK. Expression of nitric oxide synthase by syncytiotrophoblast in human placental villi. *FASEB* 1993;**7**:1269–76.

46 Morris NH, Eaton BM, Sooranna SR, Steer PJ. NO synthase activity in placental bed and tissues from normotensive pregnant women. *Lancet* 1993;**342**:679–80.

47 Ghabour MS, Eis ALW, Brockman DE, Pollock JS, Myatt L. Immunohistochemical characterization of placental nitric oxide synthase expression in preeclampsia. *Am J Obstet Gynecol* 1995;**173**:687–94.

48 Buttery LDK, McCarthy A, Springall DR *et al.* Endothelial nitric oxide synthase in the human placenta: regional distribution and proposed regulatory role at the feto-maternal interface. *Placenta* 1994;**15**:257–65.

49 Molnar M, Hertelendy F. Nω-Nitro-L-arginine, an inhibitor of nitric oxide synthesis, increases blood pressure in rats and reverses the pregnancy-induced refractoriness to vasopressor agents. *Am J Obstet Gynecol* 1992;**166**:1560–7.

50 Baylis C, Engels K. Adverse interactions between pregnancy and a new model of systemic hypertension produced by chronic blockade of endothelial-derived relaxing factor (EDRF) in the rat. *Clin Exp Hypertens Preg* 1992;**B11**:117–29.

51 Yallampalli C, Garfield RE. Inhibition of nitric oxide synthesis in rats during pregnancy produces signs similar to those of preeclampsia. *Am J Obstet Gynecol* 1993;**169**:1316–20.

52 Molnar M, Suto T, Toth T, Hertelendy F. Prolonged blockade of nitric oxide synthesis in gravid rats produces sustained hypertension, proteinuria, thrombocytopenia and intrauterine growth retardation. *Am J Obstet Gynecol* 1994;**170**:1458–66.

53 Seligman SP, Buyon JP, Clancy RM, Young BK, Abramson SB. The role of nitric oxide in the pathogenesis of pre-eclampsia. *Am J Obstet Gynecol* 1994;**171**:944–8.

54 Lyall F, Young A, Greer IA. Nitric oxide concentrations are increased in the fetoplacental circulation in preeclampsia. *Am J Obstet Gynecol* 1995;**173**:714–18.

55 Cameron IT, van Papendorp CL, Palmer RMJ, Smith SK, Moncada S. Relationship between nitric oxide synthesis and increase in systolic blood pressure in women with hypertension in pregnancy. *Hypertens Preg* 1993;**12**:85–92.

56 Davidge ST, Stranko CP, Roberts JM. Urine but not plasma nitric oxide metabolites are decreased in women with pre-eclampsia. *Am J Obstet Gynecol* 1996;**174**:1008–13.

57 Morris NH, Sooranna SR, Learmont JG *et al.* Nitric oxide synthase activities in placental tissue from normotensive, pre-eclamptic and growth retarded preg-

nancies. *Br J Obstet Gynaecol* 1995;**102**:711–14.

58 Pinto A, Sorrentino R, Sorrentino P *et al*. Endothelial-derived relaxing factor released by endothelial cells of human umbilical vessels and its impairment in pregnancy-induced hypertension. *Am J Obstet Gynecol* 1991;**164**:507–13.

59 Orpana AK, Avela K, Ranta V, Viinikka L, Ylikorkala O. The calcium-dependent nitric oxide production of human vascular endothelial cells in pre-eclampsia. *Am J Obstet Gynecol* 1996;**174**:1056–60.

60 Roberts JM, Edep ME, Goldfien A, Taylor RN. Sera from pre-eclamptic women specifically activate human umbilical vein endothelial cells *in vitro*: morphological and biochemical evidence. *Am J Reprod Immunol* 1992;**27**:101–8.

61 Taylor RN, Casal DC, Jones LA, Varma M, Martin JN, Roberts JM. Selective effects of pre-eclamptic sera on human endothelial cell procoagulant protein expression. *Am J Obstet Gynecol* 1991;**165**:1705–10.

62 Taylor RN, Musci TJ, Rodgers GM, Roberts JM. Prepartum pre-eclamptic sera stimulate platelet-derived growth factor mRNA and protein production by cultured human endothelial cells. *Am J Reprod Immunol* 1991;**25**:105–8.

63 Branch DW, Dudley DJ, LaMarche S, Mitchell MD. Sera from preeclamptic patients contain factor(s) that stimulate prostacyclin production by human endothelial cells. *Prostaglandins, Leukotrienes Essential Fatty Acids* 1992;**45**:191–5.

64 de Groot CJM, Davidge ST, Friedman SA, McLaughlin MK, Roberts JM, Taylor RN. Plasma from preeclamptic women increases human endothelial cell prostacyclin production without change in cellular enzyme activity or mass. *Am J Obstet Gynecol* 1995;**172**:976–85.

65 Gallery EDM, Rowe J, Campbell S, Hawkins T. Effect of serum on secretion of prostacyclin and endothelin–1 by decidual endothelial cells from normal and preeclamptic pregnancies. *Am J Obstet Gynecol* 1995;**173**:918–23.

66 Baker PN, Davidge ST, Barankiewicz J, Roberts JM. Plasma of pre-eclamptic women stimulates and then inhibits endothelial prostacyclin. *Hypertension* 1996;**27**:56–61.

67 Davidge ST, Baker PN, Roberts JM. NOS expression is increased in endothelial cells exposed to plasma from women with preeclampsia. *Am J Physiol* 1995;**269**:H1106-12.

68 Baker PN, Davidge ST, Roberts JM. Plasma from women with pre-eclampsia increases endothelial cell nitric oxide production. *Hypertension* 1995;**26**:244–8.

69 Baker PN, Stranko CP, Davidge ST, Davies PS, Roberts JM. Mechanical stress eliminates the effects of plasma from patients with preeclampsia on endothelial cells. *Am J Obstet Gynecol* 1996;**174**:730–6.

70 Smarason AK, Sargent IL, Redman CWG. Endothelial cell proliferation is suppressed by plasma but not serum from women with pre-eclampsia. *Am J Obstet Gynecol* 1996;**174**:787–93.

71 Chua S, Wilkins T, Sargent I, Redman C. Trophoblast deportation in pre-eclamptic pregnancy. *Br J Obstet Gynaecol* 1991;**98**:973–9.

72 Jones CJ, Fox H. An ultrastructural and ultrahistochemical study of the human placenta in maternal pre-eclampsia. *Placenta* 1980;**1**:61–76.

73 Smarason AK, Sargent IL, Starkey PM, Redman CWG. The effect of placental syncytiotrophoblast microvillous membranes from normal and pre-eclamptic women on the growth of endothelial cells *in vitro*. *Br J Obstet Gynaecol* 1993;**100**:943–9.

74 Greer IA, Haddad NG, Dawes J, Johnstone FD, Calder AA. Neutrophil activation in pregnancy-induced hypertension. *Br J Obstet Gynaecol* 1989;**96**:978–82.

75 Lyall F, Greer IA, Boswell F, Macara LM. The cell adhesion molecule VCAM–1 is selectively elevated in serum in pre-eclampsia: does this indicate the mechanism of leucocyte activation? *Br J Obstet Gynaecol* 1994;**101**:485–7.

76 Greer IA, Lyall F, Perera T, Boswell F, Macara LM. Increased concentrations of

cytokines, interleukin–6 and interleukin–1 receptor antagonist in plasma of women with pre-eclampsia: a mechanism for endothelial dysfunction. *Obstet Gynecol* 1994;84:937–40.

77 Vince GS, Starkey PM, Austgulen R, Kwiatowski D, Redman CWG. Interleukin–6, tumour necrosis factor and soluble tumour necrosis factor receptors in women with pre-eclampsia. *Br J Obstet Gynaecol* 1995;102:20–5.

78 Hubel CA, Roberts JM, Taylor RN *et al.* Lipid peroxidation in pregnancy: new perspectives on pre-eclampsia. *Am J Obstet Gynecol* 1989;161:1025–34.

79 Tsukimori K, Maeda H, Ishida K, Nagata O, Koyanagi T, Nakano H. The superoxide generation of neutrophils in normal and pre-eclamptic pregnancies. *Obstet Gynecol* 1993;81:536–40.

80 Hubel CA, McLaughlin MK, Evans RW, Hauth BA, Sims CJ, Roberts JM. Fasting serum triglycerides, free fatty acids, and malondialdehyde are increased in preeclampsia, are positively correlated, and decrease within 48 hours post partum. *Am J Obstet Gynecol* 1996;174:975–82.

81 Lorentzen B, Endersen MJ, Clausen T, Henriksen T. Fasting serum free fatty acids and triglycerides are increased before 20 weeks of gestation in women who later develop pre-eclampsia. *Hypertens Preg* 1994;13:103–9.

82 Endresen MJ, Lorentzen B, Henriksen T. Increased lipolytic activity and high ratio of free fatty acids to albumin in sera from women with pre-eclampsia leads to triglyceride accumulation in cultured endothelial cells. *Am J Obstet Gynecol* 1992;167:440–7.

83 Lorentzen B, Endresen MJ, Hovig T, Haug E, Henriksen T. Sera from preeclamptic women increase the content of triglycerides and reduce the release of prostacyclin in cultured endothelial cells. *Thromb Res* 1991;63:363–72.

84 Endresen MJ, Tosti E, Heimli H, Lorentzen B, Henriksen T. Effects of free fatty acids found increased in women who develop pre-eclampsia on the ability of endothelial cells to produce prostacyclin, cGMP and inhibit platelet aggregation. *Scand J Clin Lab Invest* 1994;54:549–57.

85 Uotila JT, Tuimala RJ, Aarnio TM, Pyykko KA, Ahotupa MO. Findings on lipid peroxidation and antioxidant function in hypertensive complications of pregnancy. *Br J Obstet Gynaecol* 1993;100:270–6.

86 Wisdom SJ, Wilson R, McKillop JH, Walker JJ. Antioxidant systems in normal pregnancy and in pregnancy-induced hypertension. *Am J Obstet Gynecol* 1991;165:1701–4.

87 Davidge ST, Hubel CA, Brayden RD, Capeless EC, McLaughlin MK. Sera antioxidant activity in uncomplicated and preeclamptic pregnancies. *Obstet Gynecol* 1992;79:897–901.

88 Garzetti GG, Tranquilli AL, Cugini AM, Mazzanti L, Cester N, Romanini C. Altered lipid composition, increased lipid peroxidation and altered fluidity of the membrane as evidence of platelet damage in preeclampsia. *Obstet Gynecol* 1993;81:337–40.

89 Galle J, Bassenge E, Busse R. Oxidized low density lipoproteins potentiate vasoconstrictions to various agonists by direct interaction with vascular smooth muscle. *Circ Res* 1990;66:1287–93.

90 Sattar N, Gaw A, Packard CJ, Greer IA. Potential pathogenic roles of aberrant lipoprotein and fatty acid metabolism in pre-eclampsia. *Br J Obstet Gynaecol* 1996;103:614–20.

6 Prediction and Prevention of Pre-eclampsia

D CHURCHILL AND DG BEEVERS

Introduction

This chapter will focus on pre-eclampsia. Indeed to concentrate upon any other hypertensive condition may miss the point, as it is pre-eclampsia and its related conditions which contribute to the majority of the morbidity and mortality associated with the hypertensive disorders in pregnancy.

Unfortunately attempts to devise an accurate predictive test for pre-eclampsia have been hindered by a lack of knowledge surrounding the aetiology of the disorder and an incomplete understanding of its pathophysiology, although important advances are currently being made. Because of these handicaps, the best that can be hoped for is to be able to identify a sub-group of women who may be more at risk of developing the disorder. With this approach it is inevitable that these groups will be somewhat heterogeneous, containing many false positives within the selection. This problem will have a negative effect on the efficiency of the screening test(s) employed. Therefore, clinicians have to be honest with both their patients and themselves when using such inherently insecure methods of screening, especially when the screening programme used may lead to a cohort of women being offered a particular treatment or plan of care. However innocuous the treatment may seem, there will always be a cost, if only in terms of the anxiety it causes to the woman herself by labelling her as an at risk individual.

The number of screening tests devised to detect or predict PET seems to be legion. Not all will be discussed in this book and readers will have to refer to other texts for a comprehensive breakdown. However some of the more practical, promising and/or successful tests will be elaborated upon in order to give the practising clinician, whether that be a midwife, GP, obstetrician or clinical researcher, some markers that can be laid down to identify at-risk women. Some other tests will be mentioned for historical interest.

Practice Point – Principles of Prevention

- Prevention of a disease or disease process first requires an intimate understanding of the aetiology or pathophysiology of that disease or process, and an effective modality of treatment. At present neither situation pertains for pre-eclampsia

---

Identifying At-risk Pregnancies

Clinical risk factors

Epidemiological research has identified several risk factors for the development of pre-eclampsia. Some have stronger associations than others, but all have a role to play in identifying women at risk of the disorder. In addition, several protective factors have also been identified, although just as possessing a risk factor does not necessarily mean that a woman will develop pre-eclampsia, neither does the absence of any risk factor guarantee safety.

Primigravidae, or more precisely nulliparae, have been known for many years to be at increased risk of developing pre-eclampsia. Even a previous miscarriage confers some protection against developing the disorder. If all primigravidae are at risk then this will include around 30% of the total pregnant population, which means with a disease incidence of between 2% to 5% the majority of women have nothing to worry about. This does not mean that these women should be ignored, merely that no undue anxiety needs to be engendered in the absence of either other risk factors or confirmatory symptoms or signs of the disease process itself.

A large case control study carried out in 1991 compared over 200 women who had suffered pre-eclampsia in a previous pregnancy, with controls who had had previous pregnancies unaffected by either hypertension or pre-eclampsia.[1] Several significant risk factors were identified which predispose an individual to the development of pre-eclampsia. These factors were: nulliparity, a previous history of pre-eclampsia, a high body mass index, physical work during pregnancy, a family history of pre-eclampsia, and an African-American ethnic background. Confirmation for some of these risk factors came in 1994, when another study also identified three of these factors as significant: severe obesity, a previous history of pre-eclampsia and a pre-pregnancy weight of > 84 kg.[2]

Other known but often-neglected risk factors include: low socio-economic status, multiple pregnancies, diabetes, hydramnios, rhesus isoimmunization, and trophoblastic disease. Pregnancies complicated by other medical diseases, such as diabetes, become highly complicated when pre-eclampsia occurs in conjunction with these other conditions. It emphasises the need for a multi-disciplinary approach towards managing these cases.

The influence of a family history of PET upon an individual's own risk of suffering from the disorder has led to many theories about the genetic origins of the condition. It was once believed that pre-eclampsia was a single gene disorder, but this belief is now on the wane. However, the strength of the association between a family history of the disease and the individual risk of contracting PET emphasises that there is some inherent genetic component to its origins. Using an average gene frequency of 0.225 in the general population, the expected incidence of pre-eclampsia would be approximately 5%, close to the observed incidence of the disease. For daughters of mothers who suffered from pre-eclampsia in their pregnancies, the incidence would rise to 22% and where a sister had suffered from pre-eclampsia this would rise further to 38%. Carefully conducted family studies have shown that the relative risk of pre-eclampsia for daughters of women who have suffered from the disorder is seven times that of the normal background risk. It is still somewhat uncertain as to whether or not these family studies are applicable to the general population.[3]

Practice Point – Risk Factors Predisposing to Pre-eclampsia

- Primigravidity
- Previous history of pre-eclampsia
- High body mass index > 27 kg/m^2
- Physical work later in pregnancy
- Family history of pre-eclampsia
- Low socioeconomic status
- Multiple pregnancies
- Diabetes mellitus
- Hydramnios
- Rhesus isoimmunisation
- Trophoblastic disease

Blood pressure measurement as a predictor

As blood pressure is fundamental to the diagnosis of pre-eclampsia, it is not surprising that many attempts have been made to harness it as an early warning sign. However, using the main diagnostic sign as a predictor in itself poses several scientific problems.

It is well known that women who develop hypertension in later pregnancy have significantly higher blood pressures in early pregnancy when compared to the rest of the pregnant population.[4,5] Unfortunately, because of the overlap between the two groups, no clear demarcation or threshold has been found which would make the blood pressure level *per se* a suitable screening test to identify a collective at-risk group. The mean arterial pressure (MAP), a derivative of the systolic and diastolic pressures,[2] has also been studied with a view to using it as a predictor of hypertension. A large prospective study found that with every 5 mmHg rise in MAP there was a progressive rise in the perinatal mortality. In the second trimester of pregnancy, a MAP of 90 mmHg or above was associated with a significant increase in the stillbirth rate, frequency of pre-eclampsia, and intrauterine growth retardation.[6] However, the number of false positive individuals included in the group was high, and like other studies the positive predictive value of the MAP is poor.

A study in 1989 of 700 normotensive women examined the MAP and threshold rises in diastolic (>15 mmHg) and systolic (>30 mmHg) blood pressures, alone and in combination, as indicative of patients being at risk of developing pre-eclampsia.[7] In the sub-group of primigravidae the true incidence of pre-eclampsia was 19.6%, substantially higher than the background incidence of the disease. Therefore there may have been some bias within their population selection. Nevertheless, the predictive values for each measurement were calculated and are shown in Table 6.1.

Table 6.1 The sensitivities and positive predictive values for the development of pre-eclampsia as determined by three measures of blood pressure

Test	Sensitivity	Positive predictive value
MAP >90 mmHg	8%	32%
Increase in diastolic pressure >15 mmHg	39%	32%
Increase in systolic pressure >30 mmHg	22%	33%

The negative predictive values for the measures ranged between 81% and 85%, with no one measure significantly better at predicting the disease. Other workers found similar results.[8]

Attempts have been made to harness the disordered vascular responsiveness, which occurs in pre-eclampsia, to predict the onset of the disease, and the "roll over" test was thus devised. The test involves measuring the blood pressure in the left lateral and then supine positions between 28 and 32 weeks' gestation. A 20 mmHg rise in diastolic pressure when the patient is rolled into the supine position had a specificity of 91% for the development of pre-eclampsia. However other measures of its screening potential were not stated. Repetition of this work failed to confirm these good results and the test fell into disuse.[9]

Clearly no measure of blood pressure is, in itself, sufficiently accurate to warrant its wholesale use as a screening tool. But in combination with other clinical risk factors it does serve to heighten awareness in certain individuals as to the possibility of their developing pre-eclampsia.

Practice Point – Prediction

- The use of blood pressure to predict a disease, in which it is fundamental to the definition, has several conceptual and scientific problems; and therefore should be treated with caution.

Doppler ultrasound

Doppler ultrasound of the **uterine** arteries has shown some merit as a predictive test for diseases such as pre-eclampsia and intrauterine growth retardation (IUGR). In a two-stage study, Doppler ultrasound of the uterine artery was performed, first between 18 and 22 weeks' gestation and then at 24 weeks' gestation. The presence of a persistent early diastolic/dichrotic "notch" (Figure 6.1) was found to be a significant predictor for pre-eclampsia.[10] Women displaying this feature were 68 times more likely to develop pre-eclampsia than their counterparts without "notching". The test had a high sensitivity and specificity of 75% and 96% respectively, however the positive predictive value was only 28%. Nevertheless, these results were promising and follow-up studies were undertaken.[11] Similar work studying waveforms in the uteroplacental circulation from both sides of the uterus found

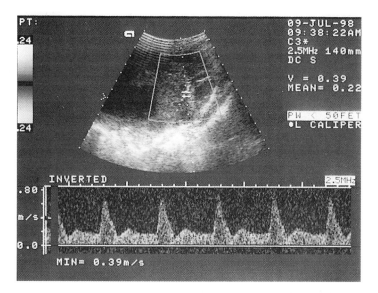

Figure 6.1 Doppler waveforms of the uterine artery showing early diastolic notching. This is predictive of a pregnancy at high risk of developing pre-eclampsia and intrauterine growth retardation.

equally good results.[12] Instead of "notching", a semi-quantitative measure, the resistance index was used as the measure from which predictions could be made. The cut-off value for the resistance index was chosen at 0.58 from previous published work. The sensitivity for hypertension alone in later pregnancy was 39%. When true pre-eclampsia was the outcome variable this rose to 63%, and for IUGR it was 100%. The positive predictive values for these conditions were 25%, 10%, and 13% respectively. The results were encouraging and it is suggested that Doppler ultrasound may be a way of selecting out high-risk pregnancies for further monitoring in the antenatal period.

A recent study using transvaginal Doppler ultrasound between 12 and 16 weeks' gestation has also demonstrated an association between bilateral uterine artery notching and the development of pre-eclampsia in later pregnancy.[13] While this confirms the previous study's findings, it also suggests that the screening can possibly be carried out even earlier in a pregnancy.

A great deal of work has and is being carried out looking at the possibilities of incorporating uterine or umbilical artery Doppler ultrasound into the fetal anomaly screening scan, usually undertaken at 18–20 weeks' gestation. Indeed it has become an accepted tool for the assessment of pregnancies known to be affected by problems such as IUGR or pre-eclampsia.[14] It would not be too surprising in the future if a screening test or procedure for both these conditions were developed using the technique of Doppler ultrasound. Further studies are needed though before its widespread introduction into clinical practice as a screening tool. There will also need to be evidence that it will be cost effective as well as clinically feasible.

Practice Point – Prediction

- To date Doppler ultrasound has shown the greatest promise as a possible screening tool to identify pregnancies at risk of pre-eclampsia and IUGR

Uric acid

Plasma uric acid is a sensitive indicator of the severity of pre-eclampsia. There is difficulty, however, in demonstrating any difference in serum uric acid levels in women with mild, moderate or severe pre-eclampsia when compared to the whole population between 36 and 40 weeks' gestation.[15] It has been suggested that the greatest benefit can be obtained in measuring the serum urate at between 24 and 32 weeks' gestation, the time of the highest fetal mortality associated with the condition.[16]

It is clear that as a predictor of pre-eclampsia, uric acid has no role to play; however, it is useful in assessing the severity of the disease once a woman has been identified as suffering from pre-eclampsia.

Fibronectin

Fibronectin is a glycoprotein present in many tissues and body fluids. The soluble form (plasma fibronectin) is present in the plasma in high concentrations. The insoluble form is called cellular fibronectin and is produced by fibroblasts, endothelium, macrophages, and blood platelets. It is also widespread in connective tissue and basement membranes. Increased levels of plasma fibronectin have been found in association with pre-eclampsia.[17] It was claimed that increased fibronectin levels predicted the development of "gestational hypertension" with a sensitivity of 96% and a

102

specificity of 94%. Unfortunately, fibronectin levels change in association with several disease states, some of which can be associated with pre-eclampsia. Levels have been found to decrease in cases of liver insufficiency, disseminated intravascular coagulopathy (DIC), respiratory distress syndrome (RDS), and sepsis, and to increase in chronic inflammatory states such as rheumatoid arthritis.

Other workers have investigated the endothelial cell derived isoform of fibronectin in the plasma.[18] Patients were studied during each of the three trimesters. No statistical difference was seen in the first trimester, but levels of fibronectin in women destined to have pre-eclampsia were higher in the second trimester than in the matched controls. Other clinical parameters such as blood pressure did not achieve clinical significance until the third trimester. The results suggested that the maternal vascular cell injury is detectable prior to the onset of the disease. However, fibronectin in general will not be useful as a predictor as there is a large overlap in values between normal and abnormal, limiting its powers of discrimination.

Angiotensin infusion test

This test is of more historical and academic interest than true practical value. It was again an attempt to harness the altered vascular responsiveness found in pre-eclampsia. Patients with pre-eclampsia are known to be hyper-responsive to the renin angiotensin system, whereas in normal pregnancies the responsiveness is markedly decreased. By infusing serial dilutions of angiotensin and observing the changes in blood pressure, it was suggested that women at greater likelihood of developing pre-eclampsia could be identified.[19] At first the results seemed very encouraging, but unfortunately could not be replicated in other studies. When added to the fact that the test was highly invasive and potentially dangerous, it was clearly never destined to be a serious widespread screening test.[20]

Microalbuminuria

Glomerular endotheliosis and the leakage of protein into the urine is characteristic of pre-eclampsia. It has been suggested that the changes in the glomerular capillary wall predate the onset of hypertension,[21] and therefore proteinuria, in the form of micro-albuminuria, may be predictive of pre-eclampsia. Results from various studies have been conflicting. One large epidemiological study found a significant association between microalbuminuria and preterm delivery but not pre-eclampsia.[22] Other studies have found both positive and negative results and have come to opposite conclusions.[23,24]

A new immunochemical dipstix test has recently been developed for the detection of microalbuminuria. Preliminary findings in a small group of women where the dipstix was used have yielded promising results. In this group of women the sensitivity for the detection of hypertension plus proteinuria or oedema was 68% and the specificity 92%, giving a positive predictive value of 56%. This method of predicting pre-eclampsia needs further evaluation in large population studies, but if it is successful it has great potential.[25]

Angiotensin II platelet binding

A significant correlation has been found between the level of angiotensin II platelet binding and the diastolic pressure in response to infusions of serial dilutions of angiotensin. Angiotensin II binding to platelets was six times higher in hypertensive women than normotensive women. More recently angiotensin II platelet receptor levels have been assayed. A correlation between the levels of receptors on platelets and blood pressure has been found. Unfortunately, a recent prospective study from China failed to show any benefit from tests of A-II receptor status in predicting hypertension in pregnancy. However, the study was contaminated in its design and was trying to test too many hypotheses at once.[26] Doubtless it will not be the last word on this subject; there is intense interest in these tests. Their predictive values are too low to stand alone as a single test and it is possible that they may need to be combined with other investigations such as Doppler ultrasound if they are to become part of a screening programme for pre-eclampsia.[27]

Urinary kallikrein : creatinine ratio

Kallikrein is excreted in the urine in both active and inactive forms. It is thought to play an important role in regulating blood pressure via the generation of vasodilatory kinins and the stimulation of prostaglandin biosynthesis.

Prospective studies have shown a lowered active and inactive kallikrein excretion, detectable prior to the rise in blood pressure, when compared to normal controls. In these studies the urine samples were timed and taken under supervision.

In order to simplify the collection and biochemical analysis using untimed spot urine samples, a test has been devised whereby active and inactive kallikrein are expressed as ratios to creatinine levels.[28] The study claimed to demonstrate that the measurement of the inactive kallikrein to creatinine ratio provided a practical means by which to assess the risk of pre-eclampsia. As a screening test its potential is still unknown, but early results suggest some promise. It certainly warrants further investigation.

Multiple parameter risk scoring

With so many tests to choose from, it is not surprising that multiple test models have been and are being investigated. The obvious problem with multiple testing of patients is that different risk factors carry different weights. Efforts have been made to produce a profile scoring system. One study used five clinical parameters – the roll over test, MAP, ocular arteriolar vasospasm, hand and facial oedema, and patellar reflexes; and eight laboratory tests – urine protein, serum urate, urea nitrogen, creatinine, albumin, total proteins, platelet count and plasma fibrinogen.[29] Values for each parameter were chosen as normal or abnormal, and, based upon the degree of abnormality, the patient was assessed for each parameter by arbitrarily giving a score for the measure. It was possible to produce a suitable risk profiling system, but the number of parameters in the profile make it unsuitable as a screening test.

Preventing the Development of Pre-eclampsia

In order successfully to prevent a particular disease process, it is usual either to know its cause, or secondly have a biological mechanism by which the disease can be detected at a subclinical level. This presupposes that a ready preventative treatment is available, but none of these requirements can be fulfilled in the case of pre-eclampsia. Of course, it is possible to prevent some diseases without knowing the cause or the mechanism by which the diseases act. The very early days of immunisation against infectious diseases are an example of this taking place. However, a lack of detailed knowledge about disease processes as complicated as pre-eclampsia severely impairs the success of the preventative measures undertaken.

Low dose aspirin

Interest in the preventative properties of low dose aspirin in pre-eclampsia stems from the knowledge of its action in preventing platelet aggregation. This is achieved by inhibiting the activity of the enzyme cyclo-oxygenase, thereby reducing the production of thromboxane, allowing the balance between thromboxane and prostacyclin to tip in favour of the latter compound. This is a powerful platelet anti-aggregator and vasodilator.[30] By acting in this way, low dose (LD) aspirin reduces the amount of intra-vascular thrombosis and endothelial damage taking place in the placenta of pre-eclamptics. Thus it is said to improve placental perfusion and by interrupting, at least in part, the vicious spiral of thrombosis and endothelial damage, reduces the "toxin" release from the placenta.

Several randomised trials of LD aspirin versus placebo were carried out in groups of patients at high risk of developing pre-eclampsia and/or IUGR.[31-34] Significant advantages were demonstrated in the groups taking aspirin. The incidence of pre-eclampsia was reduced and the birth weights of the resulting infants were higher than in the control groups. A meta-analysis of these trials suggested that the effect in the reduction of pre-eclampsia was real and significant. These findings excited many workers around the world and seemed to offer hope that a simple measure could be widely employed to prevent the worst effects of pre-eclampsia on a global scale. Several large randomised trials were then undertaken asking the same questions in large groups of women considered as being at risk of either PET or IUGR. The first two to report were the Italian[35] and American[36] multi-centre trials. There were no significant differences between the group of patients taking aspirin and the group taking placebo in the development of pre-eclampsia, birth weights of infants, and perinatal mortality. Worryingly, the American trial appeared to show an excess of placental abruption in the treatment group.

A more definitive answer regarding LD aspirin came with the publication of the CLASP trial results.[37] In this large randomised placebo controlled trial nearly 10 000 pregnant women considered to be at risk of either pre-eclampsia or IUGR, were randomised to receive either 60 mg of aspirin daily or placebo. Aspirin was associated with a 12% reduction in the incidence of pre-eclampsia, but this was not statistically significant, nor was there any significant difference in the rates of IUGR, stillbirth or neonatal death (Figures 6.2 and 6.3). Sub-group analysis did suggest that women at risk of early onset pre-eclampsia, i.e. before 32 weeks' gestation, would benefit from low dose aspirin resulting in a reduction in the incidence of pre-eclampsia. However, the numbers in the sub-groups were too small to have the power to achieve statistical significance. There was, however, no increase in the incidence of placental abruption as suggested by the earlier report from the USA.

Practice Point – Prevention

• Low dose aspirin does not increase the incidence of placental abruption

---

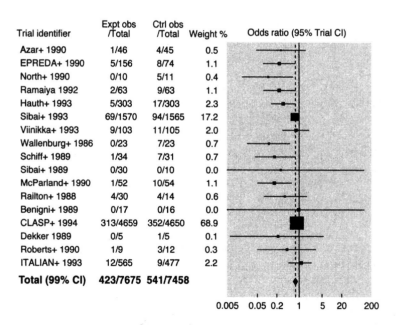

Trial identifier	Expt obs /Total	Ctrl obs /Total	Weight %	Odds ratio (95% Trial CI)
Azar+ 1990	1/46	4/45	0.5	
EPREDA+ 1990	5/156	8/74	1.1	
North+ 1990	0/10	5/11	0.4	
Ramaiya 1992	2/63	9/63	1.1	
Hauth+ 1993	5/303	17/303	2.3	
Sibai+ 1993	69/1570	94/1565	17.2	
Viinikka+ 1993	9/103	11/105	2.0	
Wallenburg+ 1986	0/23	7/23	0.7	
Schiff+ 1989	1/34	7/31	0.7	
Sibai+ 1989	0/30	0/10	0.0	
McParland+ 1990	1/52	10/54	1.1	
Railton+ 1988	4/30	4/14	0.6	
Benigni+ 1989	0/17	0/16	0.0	
CLASP+ 1994	313/4659	352/4650	68.9	
Dekker 1989	0/5	1/5	0.1	
Roberts+ 1990	1/9	3/12	0.3	
ITALIAN+ 1993	12/565	9/477	2.2	
Total (99% CI)	**423/7675**	**541/7458**		

0.005   0.05 0.2   1   5   20   200

Figure 6.2   A meta-analysis of trials of antiplatelet agents to prevent intra-uterine growth retardation and pre-eclampsia. The main outcome measure of the analysis is proteinuric pre-eclampsia. There is a general trend for the trials to be to the left of the line of unity. Overall the results show a small reduction in the incidence of PET.

Taken together, it is difficult to recommend the general use of LD aspirin as a preventative measure for pre-eclampsia. Its use in high-risk patients too has recently been called into question. The latest randomised trial of low dose aspirin examined the potential benefits of the agent in four groups of pregnant women at very high risk of PET. The groups were women with insulin dependent diabetes mellitus, women with chronic hypertension, women with multiple pregnancies and women who had had previous PET. No differences were found in the incidences of PET in either the aspirin or placebo patients in each of the four groups. This trial does not provide the definitive answer on LD aspirin, as there were certain methodological differences between it and previous trials, e.g. therapy was given only between 13 and 26 weeks' gestation. While it raises more doubts about the use of LD aspirin and the prevention of PET, it still leaves some questions to be answered.[38]

Given the weight of evidence overall and the absence of a conclusive randomised trial, it is our view that women who have

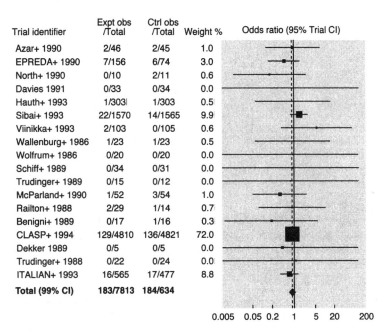

Figure 6.3 A meta-analysis of trials of antiplatelet agents to prevent IUGR and pre-eclampsia. The main outcome measure in this analysis is perinatal mortality. Overall there is no significant reduction in perinatal mortality with the use of low dose aspirin.

already suffered from early onset pre-eclampsia, or who suffer from antiphospholipid syndrome, may very well benefit from aspirin therapy.[39]

Practice Point – Prevention

- The use of low dose aspirin should be limited to women with a history of early onset pre-eclampsia in a previous pregnancy, and women with the anti-phospholipid antibody syndrome

---

Calcium supplementation

Data from epidemiological and observational studies have shown that there is an inverse relationship between calcium intake and blood pressure in pregnant women. Observational data have also suggested that the higher the level of calcium intake the greater the protection against eclampsia.[40] Furthermore, it has been shown in a randomised controlled trial that a 2 g daily supplement of calcium reduced blood pressure throughout pregnancy up to and including at term.[41] From this work it was suggested that the lowering of blood pressure was clinically significant and could lead to a twofold reduction in the incidence of "pregnancy induced hypertension". Later studies have suggested that this is genuinely the case. A study in a South American population claimed to have discovered a large reduction in the incidence of "pregnancy induced hypertension".[41] However, therein lies the problem with the results. The definition could include both pre-eclamptic patients and those suffering from gestational or latent essential hypertension. Merely by lowering the blood pressure, which calcium does, a proportion of women will be removed from the group suffering from hypertensive disease. Therefore reducing the incidence of "pregnancy induced hypertension" does not equate with a reduction in the incidence of pre-eclampsia.

A trial of 2 g of elemental calcium versus placebo was recently reported from the USA.[42] The trial enrolled 4589 nulliparous primigravid women who were randomly allocated to each arm of the trial. The treatment was given daily, until either delivery, a diagnosis of PET was made or there was a suspicion of urolithiasis. Calcium did not reduce the incidence of pre-eclampsia, the number of preterm deliveries, small for gestational age births, or fetal and neonatal deaths. From this study it would seem that elemental calcium has no benefit in preventing pre-eclampsia or any other significant adverse obstetric outcome.

Fish oils and pre-eclampsia

Studies in non-pregnant individuals have demonstrated a blood pressure lowering effect in the untreated hypertensive.[43] The effect seems to be dependent upon the dose and duration of the treatment. The active components are the n-3 fatty acids, which are thought to alter the balance between prostacyclin and thromboxane, although the exact mechanism of action is unknown.

A randomised controlled trial of fish oil treatment versus olive oil versus placebo in the third trimester of pregnancy failed to show any effect on blood pressure.[44] A lot of research interest is focusing on the role of lipids in pre-eclampsia and reports in this area are awaited with interest.

Summary

Predicting who is going to suffer from hypertension or pre-eclampsia during their pregnancy with a very high degree of certainty is nigh on impossible. It is possible though to identify a group of women more at risk of hypertension from their clinical history and features. Primigravidity, a family history of pre-eclampsia, and multiple pregnancies seem particularly strong risk factors, although many more influences may contribute smaller effects. Given the imperfections of clinical assessment it still remains the mainstay of identifying the "at risk" woman. Over the years several biochemical or biophysical tests have been tried. Some, such as Doppler ultrasound and platelet angiotensin II binding are showing some promise. However they await refinement and it is probably only when they are used in combination that their true potential will be known. Other tests, such as micro-albuminuria or urinary kallikrein to creatinine ratios, may become significant tools in the future but presently are at an earlier stage of their development.

Given that we as yet cannot predict who is going to suffer from pre-eclampsia with any accuracy, the Holy Grail of a preventative treatment also remains some way off. At one time it was thought that low dose aspirin would prove to be the answer. This was not to be and its use is now rightly restricted to those at particularly high risk of developing the disease. The popularity of other treatments such as calcium supplementation and fish oils, seems to wax and wane, and from the evidence so far, they are probably not going to be of any benefit.

Therefore, it remains for the obstetrician and midwife to be ever vigilant for pre-eclampsia and its related conditions, as the majority of cases will develop largely unannounced.

References

1 Eskenazi B, Fenster L, Sidney S. A multivariate analysis of risk factors for pre-eclampsia. *J Am Med Assoc* 1991;266:237–41.

2 Stone JL, Lockwood CJ, Berkowitz GS, Alvarez M, Lapinski R, Berkowitz RL. Risk factors for severe preeclampsia. *Obstet Gynecol* 1994;83:357–61.

3 O'Brien WF. Predicting preeclampsia. *Obstet Gynecol* 1990;75:445–52.

4 Gallery EDM, Ross M, Hunyor SN, Gyory AZ. Predicting the development of pregnancy associated hypertension. The place of standardised blood pressure measurement. *Lancet* 1977;i:1273–5

5 Moutquin JM, Rainville C, Giroux L *et al*. A prospective study of blood pressure in pregnancy: prediction of preeclampsia. *Am J Obstet Gynecol* 1985;151:191–6.

6 Page EW, Christianson R. The impact of mean arterial pressure in the middle trimester upon the outcome of pregnancy. *Am J Obstet Gynecol* 1976;125:740–5.

7 Villar MA, Sibai B. Clinical significance of elevated mean arterial blood pressure in second trimester and threshold increase in systolic or diastolic blood pressure during third trimester. *Am J Obstet Gynecol* 1989;160:419–23.

8 Ales KL, Norton ME, Druzin ML. Early prediction of antepartum hypertension. *Obstet Gynecol* 1989;73:928–33.

9 Tunbridge RDG, Donnai P. Pregnancy associated hypertension, a comparison of its prediction by roll over test and plasma noradrenaline measurement in 100 primigravidae. *Br J Obstet Gynaecol* 1983;90:1027.

10 Bower S, Bewley S, Campbell S. Improved prediction of pre-eclampsia by two stage screening of the uterine arteries using the early diastolic notch and color doppler imaging. *Obstet Gynecol* 1993;82:78–83.

11 Arduini D, Rizzo G, Romanini C, Mancuso S. Utero-placental blood flow velocity waveforms as predictors of pregnancy induced hypertension. *Eur J Obstet Gynecol Reprod Biol* 1987;26:335–41.

12 Steel SA, Pearce JM, McParland P, Chamberlain GVP. Early Doppler ultrasound screening in prediction of hypertensive disorders of pregnancy. *Lancet* 1990;335:1548–51.

13 Harrington K, Carpenter RG, Goldfrad C, Campbell S. Transvaginal Doppler ultrasound of the uteroplacental circulation in the early prediction of pre-eclampsia and intrauterine growth retardation. *Br J Obstet Gynaecol* 1997;104:674–81.

14 Fairlie FM, Moretti M, Walker JJ, Sibai BM. Determinants of perinatal outcome in pregnancy induced hypertension with absence of umbilical artery end diastolic frequencies. *Am J Obstet Gynecol* 1991;164:1084–9.

15 Obiekwe BC, Chard T, Sturdee DW, Cockrill B. Serial measurement of serum uric acid as an indicator of fetal wellbeing in late pregnancy. *J Obstet Gynecol* 1984;5:17–20.

16 Redman CWG, Beilin LJ, Bonnar J, Wilkinson RH. Plasma urate measurements in predicting fetal death in hypertensive pregnancy. *Lancet* 1976;i:1370–3.

17 Ballegeer V, Spitz B, Kieckens L, Moreau H, van Assche FA, Collen D. Predictive value of increased plasma levels of fibronectin in gestational hypertension. *Am J Obstet Gynecol* 1989;161:432–6.

18 Taylor RN, Crombleholme WR, Friedman SA, Jones LA, Casai DC, Roberts J. High plasma cellular fibronectin levels correlate with biochemical and clinical features of preeclampsia but cannot be attributed to hypertension alone. *Am J Obstet Gynecol* 1991;**165**:895–901.

19 Gant NF, Chand S, Worley RJ, Whalley PJ, Crosby UD, MacDonald PC. A clinical test useful for predicting the development of acute hypertension in pregnancy. *Am J Obstet Gynecol* 1974;**120**:1–7.

20 Kyle PM, Clark SJ, Buckley D *et al.* Second trimester ambulatory blood pressure in nulliparous pregnancy: a useful screening test for preeclampsia. *Br J Obstet Gynaecol* 1993;**100**:914–19.

21 Misiani R, Marchesi D, Tirboschi G *et al.* Urinary albumin excretion in normal pregnancy and pregnancy induced hypertension. *Nephron* 1991;**59**:416–22.

22 Perry IJ, Gosling P, Sanghera K, Churchill D, Luesley DM, Beevers DG. Urinary microalbumin excretion in early pregnancy and gestational age at delivery. *Br Med J* 1993;**307**:420–1.

23 Moller LI, Hemmingsen L, Holm J. Diagnostic value of microalbuminuria in the prediction of preeclampsia. *Am J Obstet Gynecol* 1988;**159**:1452–5.

24 Konstantin Hansen KF, Hesseldahl H, Pedersen SM. Microalbuminuria as a predictor of preeclampsia. *Acta Obstet Gynecol Scand* 1992;**71**:343–6.

25 Das V, Bhargava T, Das SK, Pandey S. Microalbuminuria: a predictor of pregnancy induced hypertension. *Br J Obstet Gynaecol* 1996;**103**:928–30.

26 Rogers MS, Hung C, Arumanayagam M. Platelet angiotensin II receptor status during pregnancy in Chinese women at high risk of developing pregnancy induced hypertension. *Gynecol Obstet Invest* 1996;**42**:88–94.

27 Baker PN, Basheer T, James DK. Maternal platelet angiotensin II binding and fetal Doppler umbilical artery waveforms. *Br J Obstet Gynaecol* 1994;**101**:1009–10

28 Millar JGB, Campbell SK, Albano JDM, Higgins BR, Clark AD. Early prediction of preeclampsia by measurement of kallikrein and creatinine on a random urine sample. *Br J Obstet Gynaecol* 1996;**103**:421–6.

29 Thurnau GR, Dyer A, Depp III R, Martin AO. The development of a profile scoring system for early identification and severity assessment of pregnancy induced hypertension. *Am J Obstet Gynecol* 1983;**146**:406–16

30 Schiff E, Peleg E, Goldenberg M *et al.* The use of aspirin to prevent pregnancy induced hypertension and lower the ratio of thromboxane A2 to prostacyclin in relatively high risk pregnancies. *N Engl J Med* 1989 **321**:351–6.

31 Wallenburg HCS, Dekker GA, Makovitz JW, Rotmans P. Low dose aspirin prevents pregnancy induced hypertension and preeclampsia in angiotensin sensitive primigravidae. *Lancet* 1986;**i**:1–3.

32 Hauth JC, Goldenberg RL, Parker R *et al.* Low dose aspirin therapy to prevent preeclampsia. *Am J Obstet Gynecol* 1993;**168**:1083–93.

33 Sibai BM, Mirro R, Chesney CM, Leffler C. Low dose aspirin in pregnancy. *Obstet Gynecol* 1989;**74**:551–7.

34 Uzan M, Beaufils M, Breart G *et al.* Prevention of preeclampsia with low dose aspirin: results of the EPREDA trial. *J Perinat Med* 1990;**18s**:116.

35 Italian Study of Aspirin in Pregnancy. Low dose aspirin in prevention and treatment of intrauterine growth retardation and pregnancy induced hypertension. *Lancet* 1993;**341**:396–400.

36 Sibai BM, Caritis SN, Thom E *et al.* Prevention of preeclampsia with low-dose aspirin in healthy, nulliparous pregnant women. *N Engl J Med* 1993;**329**:1213–18.

37 CLASP collaborative group. CLASP: a randomised trial of low dose aspirin for the prevention and treatment of preeclampsia among 9364 pregnant women. *Lancet* 1994;**343**:619–29.

38 Caritis S, Sibai B, Hauth J *et al.* Low-dose aspirin to prevent pre-eclampsia in women at high risk. *N Engl J Med* 1998;**338**:701–5.

39 Broughton-Pipkin F, Crowther C, de Sweit M *et al.* Where next for prophylaxis against preeclampsia? *Br J Obstet Gynaecol* 1996;**103**:603–7.

40 Villar J, Repke J, Belizan JM, Pareja G. Calcium supplementation reduces blood pressure during pregnancy: results of a randomized controlled clinical trial. *Obstet Gynecol* 1987;**70**:317–22.

41 Lopez-Jaramillo P, Narvez M, Weigel RM, Yepez R. Calcium supplementation reduces the risk of pregnancy induced hypertension in an Andean population. *Br J Obstet Gynaecol* 1989;**96**:648–55.

42 Levine RJ, Hauth JC, Curet LB *et al.* Trial of calcium to prevent preeclampsia. *N Engl J Med* 1997;**337**:69–75.

43 Appel LJ, Miller ER, Seidler AJ *et al.* Does supplementation of diet with fish oil reduce blood pressure? A meta analysis of controlled clinical trials. *Arch Intern Med* 1993;**153**:1429–38.

44 Dalby-Salvig J, Olsen SF, Secher NJ. Effects of fish oil supplementation in late pregnancy on blood pressure: a randomised controlled trial. *Br J Obstet Gynaecol* 1996;**103**:529–33.

7 Intensive and High Dependency Care of Hypertensive Pregnant Women

DI THOMAS

Introduction

Severe pre-eclampsia can present management challenges which may only be successfully met by facilities and expertise offered on either high dependency or intensive care units. This chapter will outline evidence on when and how this type of care should be provided.

Intensive and high dependency acute care should be considered as separate entities, at the invasive end of a spectrum of patient dependency. Both are characterised by the need for more intensive nursing and medical care and more sophisticated monitoring of vital functions, which is not available on other wards. Obstetric units supervising high-risk deliveries should have immediate access to an intensive care unit. A dedicated obstetric high dependency unit is highly desirable, although many hospitals utilise the general high dependency care provision for the whole unit when necessary. The main disadvantage of this situation is the separation from the area of expert midwifery care.

Definitions

Intensive care units

ICUs provide 24 hour, one-to-one nursing care from specially trained nursing staff. Although often the nurse : patient ratio for the unit may be somewhat in excess of this ideal, it is still a laudable nursing aim. Each unit should comprise of at least four staffed beds admitting no fewer than 200 patients per annum. In 85% of units in the UK, anaesthetists provide direct consultant supervision of the patients, but multidisciplinary involvement should be the routine in managing these patients. Dedicated trainees provide 24 hour resident cover but they should be supervised by consultants with fixed sessional commitments to the ICU.

Intensive care is appropriate for patients who require or are likely to require advanced respiratory support (such as IPPV) or those requiring support of two or more organ systems. It is also useful for patients with chronic impairment of one or more systems sufficient to severely limit their daily activity (co-morbidity) and who require support for an acute reversible failure of another organ system.[1]

Available organ system support should include artificial ventilation of the lungs, inotropic and other support for the heart, haemodialysis, haemofiltration or haemodiafiltration for renal replacement therapy, and neurological monitoring. Complications associated with the hypertensive disorders of pregnancy and thromboembolic disease constitute the two most common obstetric indications for admission to the ICU, from a range of disorders including haemorrhage, diabetes, and chest disease such as severe asthma. It was noted in the 1988–90 Confidential Enquiry into Maternal Deaths (CEMD) report, that only 76% of units had an ICU on site.[2] No significant improvement in this situation had been made by the 1991–93 survey.[3]

Obstetric patients should be admitted for intensive care when two organ systems require support or when ventilatory failure, such as with pulmonary oedema or ARDS, has occurred. In addition, pregnant or postpartum women may be admitted to an ICU if less seriously ill when no intermediate level of care exists between the ward and ICU.

Practice Point – Intensive Care

- Obstetric patients need intensive care when there is either failure in two organ systems or ventilatory failure

---

High dependency care

HDUs provide care for patients requiring support for a single organ system, but exclude those needing advance respiratory support.

It is also appropriate for patients who will benefit from more detailed observation or monitoring than can safely be provided on a general ward. Also the HDU may be used as a "step down" facility between the ICU and the ward for patients who need observation or monitoring for more than a few hours.

It normally functions with a nurse to patient ratio of 1 : 2 and does not require the exclusive services of a full time resident doctor. However, assessment from the medical team responsible for the patient is required on a regular basis.

The three usual levels of care are intensive, intermediate and minimal or self care.[4]

The HDU is part of an integrated service and defined as "a system of organising patient care in which patients are grouped together in units, depending on their need for care as determined by their degree of illness, rather than by traditional factors such as medical or surgical specialty". Obstetric HDUs tend to admit patients **only** from the obstetric population, but conform in all other respects to the concept of progressive patient care.

A recent survey of facilities for high-risk patients in consultant obstetric units in the UK revealed that only 62% had a designated and staffed postoperative recovery area and only 41% had specific obstetric high dependency beds. Some units had neither consultant anaesthetic sessions nor an anaesthetist available around the clock.[5]

The Benefits of HDU/ICU Care

It is acknowledged that women suffering pre-eclampsia or eclampsia require more intensive management than those enjoying uncomplicated peripartum periods. The unpredictable and rapid nature of progression of life-threatening complications of pre-eclampsia justify very close surveillance of this group of patients.

With current trends in the UK moving toward greater maternal choice in childbirth, the diagnosis of pre-eclampsia imposes important additional responsibilities on the midwives and doctors when discussing the diagnosis with the mother (and birth partner if present). The reasons for "inflicting" the intensive hospital-based care should be clearly explained without inducing undue anxiety. It may be difficult to explain to an asymptomatic woman the reasons for admission to a "high-tech" environment and especially the need for invasive monitoring. Both she and her partner should be sensitively introduced to the area where she will be cared for, and made to feel as comfortable as possible. Any restrictions on visits from other members of the family need to be outlined at the start.

There should be well-documented protocols for their management, including criteria for admission to HDU and ICU. A high dependency area should be sensitively organised for the management of all but the most minimally affected women.

In the Report on Confidential Enquiries into Maternal Deaths in the UK (1988–90) it was noted that there were 27 deaths due to hypertensive disorders of pregnancy and there were 14 cases of eclampsia (20 and 8 in 1991–93). Substandard care was evident in 80% of cases in both triennia and most of the criticisms might be addressed by a functioning HDU.

Failure of medical and midwifery staff to recognise early enough the significance of clinical findings and enlist senior help, and failure to monitor disease progress more closely was the main criticism of the report. Although the number and rate of deaths from the hypertensive disorders of pregnancy fell in the most recent triennium, there was only a small reduction in the number of cases where the assessors felt that care had been substandard. The immediate cause of death in eclamptic and pre-eclamptic patients over the last three triennial surveys has been due to cerebral complications (41%), predominantly intracerebral haemorrhage, and pulmonary complications (45%), notably ARDS. These statistics demonstrate the importance of good blood pressure control and heightened surveillance for the complications of severe pre-eclampsia such as pulmonary oedema, both of which are made possible by the appropriate use of an HDU.

Practice Point – Obstetric HDU

- There should be well-documented, multidisciplinary, pregnancy-specific protocols which are audited regularly

---

Admission Rate to Intensive Care and High Dependency Units from the Obstetric Population

The rate of admission to intensive care has been shown to be around 1:1000 of obstetric patients,[6] although the rate may be as high as 0.64% in hospitals taking referrals for specialist care from other centres.[7]

The rate of admission to high dependency units depends upon

local criteria but may constitute 2–3% of pregnancies complicated by pre-eclampsia. Other pregnant women further augment the HDU bed occupancy with other critical illnesses such as haemorrhage, thromboembolic disease, asthma, and diabetes mellitus.

Organisation of Obstetric High Dependency Care

Whilst there are advantages of multiple bed units, most small to medium sized obstetric services (<4000 deliveries) will only require, and be able to offer, one of these acute beds in the labour ward.

The room should be well illuminated but private. The bed should be of an approved make for intensive care with the ability to move patients into other positions, including the Trendelenburg tilt and a central break for tilting the head upwards. Delivery, however, will have to be undertaken on a delivery bed.

Adequate space should exist all around the bed and flooring should be of an easily cleaned non-porous material lending itself to aseptic precautions. At least one hand-washing basin is needed. Mains sockets and service outlets including a source of pipeline oxygen and vacuum/suction equipment should be positioned at the head of the bed or on a gantry. Backup cylinder oxygen and entonox are required. Monitoring equipment will be arranged close to the bed and may optimally be suspended from the wall or ceiling. It is possible with modern monitoring equipment to create a less "clinical" environment so desired of by pregnant women. One or more intravenous fluid stands will be needed, as will at least two volumetric intravenous infusion pumps and syringe drivers. These are essential for accurate assessment of hourly fluid intake and precise titration of intravenous medication.

Nursing "stations" with a chair and large desk/lectern, and facilities for drug and intravenous fluid storage are needed. A full range of resuscitation drugs and equipment should be readily available in the room.

The charts on which the patient's observations are recorded should be at the bedside, readily accessible to the medical and nursing/midwifery staff but out of sight of the patient. An example of such a chart is shown in Figure 7.1. Each midwifery shift should comprise at least one member of staff with high dependency training and experience. The medical cover includes an on-site specialist registrar obstetrician and an anaesthetist, each supervised on a 24 hour basis by consultants in these specialties. Protocols for management of pre-eclampsia and other indications for HDU care should be developed locally and be available in the unit at all times.

The Management of the Pre-eclamptic Patient in HDU and ICU

Severe pre-eclampsia is a progressive disease with a very variable mode of presentation and rate of progression. The features of the disease are best demonstrated in relation to the normal physiological changes of pregnancy.

Physiological changes in normal pregnancy

All organ systems are affected by the developing pregnancy and the following is a summary for each system.

Cardiovascular system

The cardiac output is increased by as much as 40%, as a result of a rise in both the heart rate and stroke volume. The systemic vascular resistance and pulmonary vascular resistance are reduced by approximately 20–30%. The maternal blood volume increases, peaking at 40% above non-pregnant values, in the third trimester, but the red cell mass increases to a lesser degree, resulting in an overall 10% reduction in the haematocrit.

The central venous and pulmonary artery wedge pressure are usually unchanged. Multiple pregnancies may exaggerate further these cardiovascular changes, as will labour and delivery. It has been observed and should be noted that many of the measured cardiovascular parameters vary with posture, most notably following vena-caval compression by the gravid uterus in the supine position.

Respiratory system

In normal pregnancy there are changes in the mucosa of the upper airway which cause oedema, hyperaemia, and increased tissue friability. Diaphragmatic function is maintained in spite of upward displacement by the gravid uterus. The lateral dimensions of the thoracic cage are increased, and the ribs occupy a more horizontal position.

Of the measured and calculated lung volumes, the functional residual capacity (FRC) is reduced by 10% although the vital capacity is frequently unchanged. Overall lung compliance remains

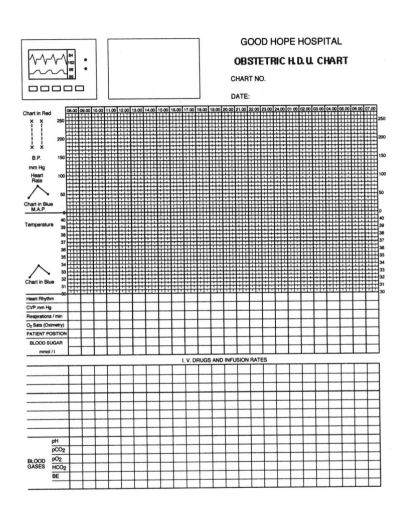

Figure 7.1 A high dependency monitoring chart used to plot the vital functions and trends in blood pressure, fluid balance, oxygen saturation, drug requirements etc.

DATE OF ADMISSION	CONSULTANT
SOURCE	MIDWIFE
DATE OF DISCHARGE	ALLERGIES
DIAGNOSIS	

FLUID BALANCE

		INTAKE														URINE OUTPUT				
														RT	HRLY	RT	NG			
	ORAL	CRYSTALLOID	COLLOID	BLOOD	HARTMANN	MgSO4	IV ANTIBIOTICS													
08.00																				
09.00																				
10.00																				
11.00																				
12.00																				
13.00																				
14.00																				
15.00																				
16.00																				
17.00																				
18.00																				
19.00																				
20.00																				
21.00																				
22.00																				
23.00																				
24.00																				
01.00																				
02.00																				
03.00																				
04.00																				
05.00																				
06.00																				
07.00																				
TOTAL INTAKE							TOTAL OUTPUT							24 HOUR BALANCE						

PUPIL SIZE		DATE OF LINE CHANGES	URINALYSIS GLUCOSE	BILIRUBIN	KETONES	S.G.	BLOOD	pH	PROTEIN	UROBILINOGEN	NITRATE
1 2	① ARTERIAL LINE										
3	② C.V.P.		X RAYS								
4	③ I.V.I.										
5	④ DRESSINGS		SPECIMENS SENT								
6	⑤ VENFLON										
7	⑥ URINARY CATHETERS										
8	⑦ NGT										

Figure 7.1   continued.

Table 7.1 CO_2 changes in pregnancy

	Normal	Pregnancy
CO_2	35–45 mmHg	28-32 mmHg
HCO_3	24 mM/l	18–21 mEq/l
pH	7.35–7.45	7.4–7.47

unchanged, although the compliance of the chest wall is reduced late in the third trimester.

Minute ventilation has increased by 20–30% at term, in response to increased metabolic production of carbon dioxide (CO_2) and also by the effect of progesterone increasing the respiratory drive. The majority of the increase in minute ventilation is achieved by an increase in tidal volume.

The arterial CO_2 level is reduced (as respiratory alkalosis) but this is partially compensated for by renal bicarbonate excretion (Table 7.1).

The arterial pO_2 is usually maintained but the reduced FRC decreases the reserve, and the pregnant woman will become desaturated more quickly with hypoventilation.

Renal physiology

Renal blood flow and glomerular filtration rate increase and the normal serum creatinine in pregnancy is lower than the usual baseline at 0.5–0.7 mg/dl (45–60 μmol/l).

Gastrointestinal physiology

The tone in the lower oesophageal sphincter is reduced in pregnancy, reaching its nadir by the 36th week. The stomach is displaced upwards by the gravid uterus and the intragastric pressure is increased further, reducing the barrier pressure (lower oesophageal pressure minus intragastric pressure). This increases the incidence of oesophageal regurgitation, and heartburn is often reported in the third trimester. The basal pH of the gastric contents is usually unchanged, but gastric emptying is delayed particularly in later pregnancy. This is exacerbated further by the use of opioid drugs in labour.

Pathophysiology of pre-eclampsia

The pathophysiological disturbances of pre-eclampsia covered in previous chapters may now be interpreted in the context of normal pregnancy, rather than by reference to the non-pregnant state. The following aspects are of particular interest for HDU/ICU management of patients.

Cardiovascular system

An increase in the systolic and diastolic blood pressure is the most obvious sign of pre-eclampsia and the change is particularly significant when related to the usual pre-pregnancy or first trimester pressure. The latter are often lower than in the non-pregnant state.

There is an exaggerated response to adrenaline and noradrenaline and increased sensitivity to angiotensin II. The cardiac index (cardiac output per square metre body surface area) is low or normal, systemic vascular resistance (SVR) normal to very high, and pulmonary capillary wedge pressure (PCWP), which is an indicator of left atrial pressure, low or normal. In severe pre-eclampsia there can be a significant disparity between the central venous pressure and the pulmonary capillary wedge pressure. In addition plasma volume may be lower, even than is found in the normal term pregnant patient.

Practice Point – Monitoring

- In severe PET there can be a significant disparity between the CVP and PCWP

Respiratory system

Pulmonary oedema is an uncommon complication of pre-eclampsia/eclampsia with an incidence of 2.9%. It occurs most commonly in association with multiple system dysfunction. Seventy per cent of episodes of pulmonary oedema occur following delivery when large changes in the balance between intravascular and extravascular fluid are still occurring. The cause is often a combination of reduced colloid osmotic pressure, increased hydrostatic pressure and increased capillary permeability.

Renal system

There is often non-selective proteinuria. This includes the passage of larger proteins such as transferrin and globulins. Most women with pre-eclampsia have mild to moderate reductions in the renal blood flow and the glomerular filtration rate. Serum creatinine therefore increases, although it should be remembered that the reference ranges for creatinine in pregnancy are lower than in the non-pregnant state and high values can be mistaken as normal.

Coagulation

Thrombocytopenia is common, occurring in about 50% of patients with PET. Significant thrombocytopenia, a platelet count $<100 \times 10^9/l$, occurs in only 15% of women with severe PET. Platelet activation is suggested by the inverse relationship between platelet count and fibrin degradation products, increased platelet-specific protein β thromboglobulin, and a reduced platelet content of serotonin (5HT). Haemolysis may occur particularly in association with abnormal liver function tests, as seen in the HELLP syndrome.

Thrombelastography (TEG) has been advocated as the most useful *in vitro* test of adequate haemostasis and the K-time and maximum amplitude variables have been shown to correlate well with the platelet count.[8] The bleeding time bears little relation to either TEG or the platelet count. From a study of 49 pre-eclamptic patients,[8] it is suggested that a platelet count of $75 \times 10^9/l$ is usually associated with normal haemostasis. The platelet count itself, and the interpretation of the TEG, is an unreliable guide to coagulation when there is abnormal interaction between platelets and vascular endothelium, as may occur in the uraemic patient or in those taking aspirin.

Indications for HDU or ICU Care in Pre-eclampsia

Any woman in whom the diagnosis of severe pre-eclampsia has been made should be managed entirely as an inpatient, and monitored in the acute phase in a designated high dependency area. As a minimum standard, intensive expert nursing/midwifery care should be available. Evidence has been presented indicating that early recognition of complications affects outcome. The main problem has always been identifying the group of patients for whom serious complications are most likely to occur. It is known that serious sequelae such as eclamptic fits can occur in the absence of significant changes in systemic arterial blood pressure; it is also known that good control of hypertension when present does not eliminate the risk of fits.

However, observations of trends in monitored parameters and the clinical features of pre-eclampsia should be expected to provide an earlier warning of treatable complications. Symptoms such as headache, irritability, and abdominal pain, and clinical signs such as hyper-reflexia and clonus, should command special attention.

Practice Point – Management

- Patients with severe pre-eclampsia should be managed by senior clinicians and midwives experienced in treating the disorder and its complications

---

Monitoring of values and trends in vital signs in the cardio-respiratory system as well as the renal output is key to pre-emptive management. It is also appropriate to follow haematological parameters, such as the platelet count, clotting function, and more specific tests, when indicated. The actual indications for admission should form the first part of the protocol for management on the HDU and an example is shown at the end of the chapter.

The decision to transfer from high dependency to intensive care is usually taken after consultation between the clinicians involved in management and is precipitated by the need for more advanced monitoring or treatment. Common examples of these include refractory eclampsia, the need for artificial ventilation, cardio-vascular instability, the need for pulmonary artery catheters, and renal insufficiency requiring haemofiltration or haemodialysis. Unlike other admissions to intensive care, this group of patients may have the additional complication of an unborn child. However, the vast majority will be delivered by the time they reach ICU.

Vital Function Monitoring in the HDU

The HDU charts facilitate the clear presentation of all the observations made and each variable may easily be related to another. It should be emphasised again that *trends* in readings from the monitoring often have greater significance than the absolute values.

Basic observations

Sophisticated monitoring should not detract from the impor-tance of clinical observation, such as skin colour, texture and temperature, and other variables such as the rate and pattern of respiration. Observations of the presence and character of deep tendon reflexes are relevant in pre-eclampsia. New findings in fundoscopy and symptoms such as headache and abdominal pain should be noted and acted upon promptly.

Cardiovascular parameters

The ECG may be displayed continuously in the HDU and ICU and, when expertly interpreted, will be an early signal of arrhythmias or ischaemia. Monitoring lead II is appropriate to identify arrhythmias but may only show signs of ischaemia occurring in the inferior part of the left ventricle. If there is any doubt, a 12 lead ECG should be performed.

Heart rate and arterial blood pressure (however measured) should be charted at least hourly. The correct cuff size should be used for patients with obese arms. The patient should be positioned correctly so that the cuff is at the same level as the heart. Undelivered patients should be lying on their left side with 30° of lateral tilt to prevent uterine pressure on the great vessels.

The Dinamap or similar automatic blood pressure measurement device may under-read the diastolic pressure when compared with manual readings. The direct methods of measurement, such as via a cannula in the radial artery, have also been shown to read lower than the sphygmomanometer by an average of 12 mmHg.[9] Automatic blood pressure readings should occasionally be checked with intermittent manual readings.

Direct arterial monitoring has the advantage of being displayed continuously (Figure 7.2), and allows access for regular haematological investigations without repeated venepuncture. The line must be regularly (or continuously) flushed and checked for damping. It should be zeroed with the transducer at the level of the heart for the pressure readings to be accurate. It should also be noted that the heparinised flush in the line may interfere with the coagulation studies performed on blood samples taken from the arterial line and the first 2 ml of any sample should be discarded.

In situations where there is uncertainty about the status of the patient's intravascular volume, or when drugs need to be given into a large vein, a central venous pressure line may offer useful additional information and access. Caution should be exercised when inserting the catheter via the internal jugular vein. The subclavian route is best avoided in the pre-eclamptic population because of the high incidence of bleeding disorders. These

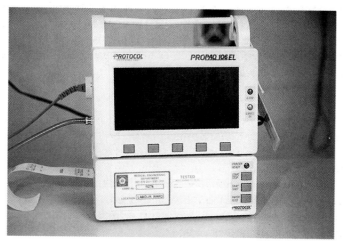

Figure 7.2 A Propaq 106 EL monitor. This portable machine can be used to monitor all vital functions and signs including intra-arterial pressure, central venous pressure and pulmonary capillary wedge pressures.

problems may be overcome by inserting a long line via the antecubital fossa.

The central venous pressure should be displayed continuously and recorded hourly on the HDU chart.

Urine output

Documentation of urine output provides additional indirect information on cardiovascular and renal performance. The volume produced for each hour should be recorded on a fluid balance chart together with an accurate assessment of input.

Arterial oxyhaemoglobin saturation

Pulse oximetry changes will reflect changes in cardiac output as well as respiratory compromise and alterations in the inspired oxygen concentration.

Temperature

The patient's temperature (axillary, oral or possibly rectal) should be recorded every hour and similarly charted.

Respiratory variables

Respiratory rate is the easiest clinical measure to record, but investigations reflecting gas transfer, such as blood gas analysis, have an important role in identifying deteriorations in respiratory function. These are seen most notably with pulmonary oedema and adult respiratory distress syndrome (ARDS).

Biochemical surveillance

Serum and urinary electrolytes, urea and creatinine, and liver function tests are performed on a daily basis as a minimum during critical phases of the illness.

Haematology

The haemoglobin, white count (including differential), platelet count, and clotting studies, such as INR and PTT, may need to be performed more frequently than daily, especially after the development of the HELLP syndrome or DIC.

Blood gases

These may easily be performed using heparinised syringes and taken either from intermittent arterial puncture or ideally from the indwelling arterial line. In addition to observation of trends in the pO_2 and pCO_2, a worsening metabolic acidosis will reflect serious deterioration and decompensation.

Treatment Protocols

Treatment is largely "symptomatic" but special attention is paid to the control of arterial blood pressure and the reduction of the risk of convulsions. The definitive treatment is always delivery of the fetoplacental unit.

Magnesium sulphate has been accepted as the mainstay of therapy elsewhere, most notably in the United States, and has recently been adopted in units in the United Kingdom following the report of the Collaborative Eclampsia Trial.[10] This clinical study has demonstrated the superiority of magnesium sulphate in preventing further convulsions after the first fit. The evidence only supports the use of magnesium after an eclamptic convulsion but many units are using the drug earlier in severe pre-eclampsia.

Management protocols should be developed for each obstetric unit (and possibly on a national basis if agreement could be reached). These should be reviewed regularly and patient outcome audited.

Example of a high dependency protocol

Women with the diagnosis of pre-eclampsia are usually managed as inpatients. They may already have been commenced on methyldopa, labetolol or nifedipine. The alpha-blocking effects of labetolol may be beneficial to the uteroplacental vasculature but there is concern that the beta-effects of this and other drugs may compromise the fetus's ability to cope with intrauterine stress.

HDU admission criteria

Any of the following will warrant admission:

- Severe refractory hypertension (systolic > 170, diastolic > 110).
- Significant hyper-reflexia, clonus, headaches or visual disturbance, or eclampsia.
- Deterioration in the clotting studies leading to a coagulopathy/ DIC.
- Liver failure, or abdominal pain from hepatic capsular stretch.
- Renal failure.

Management guidelines

Observations

1 Pulse and blood pressure measured and recorded every 30 minutes initially, but later tailored to condition of the patient.
2 Fluid balance chart, including all intake of fluids, e.g. drug diluents etc., and the hourly urine output.
3 Inspect the retinae daily.
4 Check the reflexes and look for clonus at least twice daily.
5 Auscultate the patient's chest twice daily.
6 Pulse oximetry: look for decreasing trends and investigate any desaturation below 94%.

Investigations

The following blood tests should be performed daily and more frequently for critically ill patients:

- FBC.
- PT and APTT if platelets less than 100.
- XDPs and fibrinogen if the PT/APTT are found to be abnormal.

- U&Es, creatinine and urate.
- LFTs, albumin and total proteins.

Consider the following to detect underlying medical conditions:

- Antithrombin III, protein C and S levels, lupus anticoagulant, anti-cardiolipin antibody, von Willebrand factor and 24 hour urine for metanephrines.

Initial HDU management

1 14 or 16-G venous access, consider oxygen via facemask.
2 Begin HDU chart, including parameters above (Figure 7.1).
3 Fluid therapy remains controversial but baseline crystalloid at 1–2 ml/kg per hour is then titrated to the patient's requirements in order to maintain her in fluid balance. Human albumin solution may be given for low colloid osmotic pressure but care must be taken not to cause extracellular fluid overload in severe disease.
4 If in doubt on volume status in the presence of oliguria, CVP monitoring may be indicated. Pulmonary arterial flotation catheter may be required in severe pre-eclampsia when CVP and PCWP do not always correlate.

Antihypertensive therapy

The patient may already have started therapy; however if the control is inadequate, i.e. a systolic pressure >170 mmHg, or a diastolic pressure >105 mmHg, consider the insertion of a radial arterial cannula and start:

1 oral nifedipine 10–20 mg followed by the same dose every 8 hours (not if the patient is in labour);
or
2 intravenous hydralazine as an initial bolus of 5 mg repeated as necessary every 15 minutes until control is achieved. Infusion at a rate of 4–20 mg/hour 60–300 μg/kg/hour).
3 Treat reflex tachycardia caused by either of the above with labetalol (combined alpha- and beta-blocker) 200 mg orally or 40 mg slow IV bolus, then 200 mg orally b.d. Oxyprenolol has been used with some success in this situation in a dose of 40–160 mg daily.
4 Avoid ergometrine in management of the third stage.

Anticonvulsant treatment

An eclamptic fit is an emergency. The main dangers apart from trauma are desaturation/hypoxia of the mother and fetus and aspiration of the stomach contents. Call for senior help including an anaesthetist, immediately. Assess the airway, breathing, and circulation, give oxygen, and place the patient in the lateral position. Treat the convulsion with magnesium sulphate.

Once the seizure has been controlled, start maintenance treatment with magnesium sulphate, which has been shown to be superior in the prevention of recurrent fits.

IV and IM magnesium regimes have been devised. The loading dose often causes nausea, vomiting and flushing.

Loading	4 g IV or 5 g IM in each buttock
	4–6 g IV bolus
Maintenance	5 g IM every 4 hours
	or
	1–2 g/hour intravenous infusion

Monitor the following:

- Respiration rate (>16 per minute).
- Urine output (>0.5 ml/kg/h).
- The presence of knee jerk or biceps reflexes.
- ECG, particularly for the first hour after load dose. A lengthening S–T interval is abnormal.
- Pulse oximetry.
- Mg levels for patients with signs of toxicity or recurrent fits.
- The therapeutic range = 2–4 mmol/l (4–8 mg/dl).

On the standard regime, a significant proportion of the measured serum levels will be "subtherapeutic". Signs of toxicity start with loss of reflexes, weakness, somnolence, flushing, double vision, and slurred speech. Respiratory depression or arrest occurs at around 7 mmol/l and cardiac arrest at more than 12 mmol/l. Calcium gluconate 1 g intravenously should be available in the room as an antidote to magnesium toxicity.

Magnesium is renally excreted and therefore the dose of magnesium sulphate should be reduced if the urine output falls below 0.5 ml/kg/h for 4 hours or if the urea increases to >10 mmol/l. In these cases magnesium levels should be measured at least twice daily.

Refractory seizures may require the airway to be secured with an endotracheal tube and general anaesthesia induced using thiopentone and suxamethonium. The pregnancy-associated changes, which increase the risks of regurgitation, make airway management in this situation more difficult if aspiration of the gastric contents is to be avoided.

If this level of resuscitation is necessary, the fetus needs to be delivered as a matter of urgency, if not already delivered, and intensive care management is indicated even if it has been possible to extubate the patient after control of the seizures has been obtained.

Other drugs and management issues

High-risk patients once identified should be kept nil-by-mouth, and ranitidine 150 mg given every 12 hours to reduce the volume and increase the pH of residual gastric contents. Thromboembolic prophylaxis should be administered unless the coagulation is already deranged. TED stockings should be fitted to every patient.

Analgesia

Analgesia in the form of opiates is appropriate. However, the labouring pre-eclamptic patient should probably enjoy the benefits of epidural or combined spinal/epidural block. A regional analgesic will avoid the large swings in blood pressure seen with painful contractions.

Caesarean Section

The best choice of anaesthesia for caesarean section is epidural regional anaesthesia built up slowly with the local anaesthetic combined with an opiate. Caution must be exercised with a rapid onset autonomic block, most notably with a spinal anaesthesia (subarachnoid block), causing vasodilatation in an already hypovolaemic woman.[11] Careful pre-loading with fluid is necessary before siting the block.

The main disadvantage of general anaesthesia for caesarean section in the pre-eclamptic patient is the profound rise in blood pressure following intubation. Various techniques have been advocated for avoiding this response, including the administration of lignocaine and short acting opiates such as alfentanyl, but the paediatrician should be alerted to the effects these agents may have on the newborn, e.g. respiratory depression.

Sedative drugs used in the ICU and HDU

There is a risk of obtunding protective airway reflexes, which may lead to aspiration of gastric contents in a patient whose trachea is not intubated. It should be remembered that the fetus will receive a variable concentration of these drugs and is more sensitive to any respiratory depressant effects.

Midazolam has been shown to cross the placenta less readily than diazepam, and may be a better choice of benzodiazepine. Morphine, pethidine, and fentanyl, are acceptable alternatives.

Non-depolarising muscle relaxants are used in the short term by the anaesthetist during a caesarean section under general anaesthesia, and rarely used in the intensive care unit. Muscle relaxants cross the placenta in very small amounts and are unlikely to cause clinical effects in the fetus in undelivered patients.

Inotropic agents used in the ICU

Inotropic agents may have detrimental effects on the fetus. In animal models both increases and decreases in uterine blood flow have been seen with the use of dopamine, dobutamine, adrenaline, and noradrenaline. Ephedrine is the only drug in this group found to increase maternal blood pressure and increase uterine blood flow.

The Food and Drug Administration in the United States has categorised many commonly used drugs in relation to their safety in pregnancy (Table 7.2).

Practice Point – Management

- Regional anaesthesia is preferable to general anaesthesia for patients with severe PET undergoing an operative delivery

---

Summary

The organisation of intensive care services and the provision of high dependency care are essential to the safe management of patients with severe pre-eclampsia. The success of these facilities will depend on input from experienced midwifery and nursing staff, and supervision by senior medical staff in the specialties of obstetrics, anaesthetics, and paediatrics.

Treatment protocols should be followed, with the aim of controlling the blood pressure, preventing eclampsia and the other

Table 7.2 Safety of drugs used in the ICU, according to the FDA classification of drug safety in pregnancy

Categories A & B	Category C	Category C	Categories D & X
Amphotericin	Acyclovir	Heparin	ACE inhibitors
Cephalosporins	Albuterol	Hydralazine	Tetracyclines
Cimetidine	Aminoglycosides	Labetalol	Coumadin
Clindamycin	Atracurium	Metronidazole	Acetylsalicylic acid
Erythromycin	Atropine	Midazolam	
Glycopyrrolate	Bretylium	Nifedipine	
Insulin	Benzodiazepines	Nitroglycerine	
Lidocaine (lignocaine)	Beta-blockers	Nitroprusside	
Magnesium (sulphate	Dantrolene	Pancuronium	
Meperidine	Digoxin	Phenytoin	
Naloxone	Haloperidol	Prednisolone	
Penicillins	Inotropes	Procainamide	
Propofol	Flumazenil	Suxamethonium	
Ranitidine	Fluconazole	Thiopental	
Terbutaline	Frusemide	Vercuronium	
		Vancomycin	

Categories A & B represent drugs for which no fetal risk has been demonstrated in human and/or animal studies.
Category C represents drugs in which animal studies have demonstrated adverse effects or inadequate data exists.
Categories D & X represent drugs in which evidence of human fetal risk exists.
Source: Am J Respir Crit Care Med 1995;152:417–55

complications of this disease. Participation in national and local audit of services and patient outcome should occur and it may be appropriate to work towards a nationally adopted set of guidelines for management of the hypertensive diseases of pregnancy.

References

1 *Standards for Intensive Care Units.* The Intensive Care Society. May 1997.
2 *Report on Confidential Enquiries into Maternal Deaths in the United Kingdom 1988–1990.* London: HMSO, 1994.
3 *Report on Confidential Enquiries into Maternal Deaths in the United Kingdom 1991–1993.* London: HMSO, 1994.
4 *Churchill's Medical Dictionary.* New York, Edinburgh etc.: Churchill Livingstone, 1989.
5 Cordingley JJ, Rubin AP. A survey of facilities for high risk women in consultant obstetric units. *Int J Obstet Anaesth* 1997;6:156–60.
6 Graham SG, Luxton MC. The requirement for intensive care support for the pregnant population. *Anaesthesia* 1989;44:581–4.
7 Umo-Etuk J, Lumley J, Holdcroft A. Critically ill parturient women and admission to intensive care: a five year review. *Int J Obstet Anaesth* 1996;5:79–84.
8 Orlikowski CEP, Rocke DA, Murray WB *et al.* Thrombelastography changes in pre-eclampsia and eclampsia. *Br J Anaesth* 1997;77:157–61.

9 Ginsbert J, Duncan S. Direct and indirect blood pressure measurements in pregnancy. *J Obstet Gynaecol Br Commonw* 1969;76:705.

10 Eclampsia Collaborative Group. Which anticonvulsant for women with eclampsia? Evidence from the Collaborative Eclampsia Trial. *Lancet* 1995;343:1455–63.

11 Lindemayer MD, Katz AI. Pre-eclampsia: pathophysiology, diagnosis, and management. *Ann Rev Med* 1989;40:233–50.

8 Hypertension Complicating Other Medical Conditions in Pregnancy

DG BEEVERS AND D CHURCHILL

Introduction

A blood pressure of 140/90 mmHg or more occurs at some time in pregnancy in about 10% of women. It is most likely to occur in older mothers who have had more than three previous pregnancies. It is also relatively more common in primigravidae. In approximately one-quarter of these women, the hypertension is longstanding, albeit often undiagnosed, until antenatal clinic attendance. Amongst these longstanding hypertensives the underlying diagnosis is essential hypertension in around 95% of cases. The management of these patients is discussed in detail in (Chapter 4). Hypertension may, however, complicate a great many other medical conditions which may be present in pregnancy. The most common problems are diabetes mellitus and the intrinsic renal diseases. These conditions and other rarer causes of high blood pressure are the focus of this chapter.

Diabetes Mellitus

Although there is considerable overlap, the two forms of diabetes (insulin dependent and non-insulin dependent) do differ in their aetiology, pathogenesis, and treatment. In pregnancy there is the additional syndrome of gestational diabetes. All diabetic patients should be referred to a specialist joint diabetic/obstetric clinic for careful nursing, midwifery, medical, and dietetic supervision. Many will also have raised blood pressure requiring antihypertensive therapy.

Insulin dependent (type I) diabetes mellitus (IDDM)

Almost all patients with IDDM will be receiving long term insulin therapy. Many will have either incipient or overt microangiopathy with renal and/or retinal involvement. Before the development of clinically evident diabetic nephropathy, many patients have raised levels of microalbuminuria (urine protein 30–300 mg daily) with negative urinary dipstix testing. At this stage they may have hyperfiltrating glomeruli, supra-normal creatinine clearances, and low serum creatinine levels. There is, however, good evidence that the presence of microproteinuria is a powerful predictor of the future development of overt nephropathy.[1] At this stage, hypertension becomes common in diabetic patients. It is mainly due to activation of the renin–angiotensin system with possibly a small component related to fluid volume retention.

Pregnant patients with all types of diabetes have a high incidence of stillbirth, intrauterine death, macrosomia (large babies), pre-eclampsia and congenital malformations.[2] It is usual to attempt to secure excellent control of blood glucose levels, often with a short stay in the day assessment unit or diabetic day centre in order to titrate the insulin dosages.

In the non-pregnant state there is an increasing trend to prescribe angiotensin converting enzyme (ACE) inhibitors. These drugs have been shown in several studies to delay the onset of diabetic nephropathy and reduce both proteinuria and microproteinuria.[3] This effect is independent of any reduction of blood pressure and greater than that seen with other classes of antihypertensive medication. The ACE inhibitors selectively dilate the post-glomerular efferent arterioles, leading to a reduction in intraglomerular pressure and reduced glomerular damage. For this reason, many clinicians are now opting to use ACE inhibitors in proteinuric diabetics even if their blood pressures are not raised. Similarly, there is a trend to use these drugs in patients with non-insulin dependent diabetes, even though as yet there is little secure trial evidence of protection of the kidneys in such patients. Furthermore, diabetologists are now tending to regard 140/80 mmHg as the appropriate threshold for starting antihypertensive drugs in diabetic patients. The result of these trends is that a very large proportion of patients with both forms of diabetes are likely to be receiving blood pressure lowering drugs (and particularly the ACE inhibitors) before or in the early stages of pregnancy. This trend is likely to increase further with the publication of a paper in 1998 which suggested that the ACE inhibitors can bring about a significant delay in the progression of diabetic retinopathy as well as nephropathy.[4]

Pathophysiology

- Hypertension in diabetic patients with nephropathy is due to activation of the renin–angiotensin system

---

Despite the proven long term advantages of ACE inhibitors in patients with IDDM, these agents remain absolutely contraindicated in pregnancy. Their use is associated with neonatal anuria and renal failure, oligohydramnios and some fetal developmental defects.[5]

Many women with diabetes who are of childbearing age will now be receiving these drugs. They need to be advised of the need to avoid conception, and if they wish to become pregnant they should be changed to alternative antihypertensive drugs. However, women who do conceive whilst receiving ACE inhibitors can be reassured that if these drugs are discontinued early in pregnancy and where necessary other agents are substituted, then the outcome of the pregnancy may not be adversely affected.[6] They can also be reassured that the short term discontinuation of ACE inhibitors during pregnancy does not cause any long term harm for their own health. Once pregnancy and breast-feeding are completed ACE inhibitors may be restarted.

The drugs of first choice in diabetics with hypertension are the same as in the non-diabetic state. Methyldopa, labetalol and possibly oxyprenolol are safe, and in severe resistant hypertension, nifedipine or hydralazine may be added. Atenolol is best avoided, as there are now three studies which suggest that this drug is associated with intrauterine growth reduction.[7]

Practice Point – Drugs

- ACE inhibitors are absolutely contraindicated in pregnancy and should be substituted with a more acceptable drug

Non-insulin dependent (type 2) diabetes mellitus (NIDDM)

This form of diabetes is largely a problem with older patients so it is less often encountered in pregnancy. Both microangiopathy (renal and retinal damage) and macroangiopathy, with large vessel damage, are seen. The majority of patients are also overweight. Hypertension is found in 70% of these patients and is less likely to be due to renal damage with alteration of the renin system. Total body water and sodium are increased and circulating renin and angiotensin levels are usually low.[8]

An important factor in patients with NIDDM is the presence of obesity with an associated increase in arm circumference. This can lead to serious overestimations of blood pressure unless an appropriately large arm cuff is used. If the conventional "adult" cuff, with an internal bladder measuring 12.5 cm × 23 cm is used, the systolic and diastolic pressures may be overestimated by as much as 10 mmHg in obese patients.[9]

It is best to avoid orally active antidiabetic agents in pregnancy as their use may lead to fetal hypogylcaemia. There are no long term data available on their safety or efficacy in pregnancy. All patients should be transferred to insulin therapy immediately pregnancy is diagnosed. The rules for any antihypertensive drugs that are considered necessary are the same as for IDDM; the beta-blocker atenolol is best avoided and ACE inhibitors are absolutely contraindicated. Furthermore, the use of thiazide diuretics, even in low dose, is not recommended as they may cause worsening of glucose intolerance. They should certainly not be used in pre-eclampsia where there is intravascular volume depletion and reduced uteroplacental blood flow.

Whilst dietary control in obese patients with NIDDM is recommended and may help to control the blood pressure, extreme or very rigid diets should be avoided in view of the risk of fetal undernutrition. Salt restriction may be hazardous as this may increase plasma renin and angiotensin levels. Patients should avoid an inordinately high salt diet and excessive weight gain. This can best be achieved by restricting intake of processed foods, salt snacks, and prepared meat products (e.g. sausages and hamburgers). Instead, fresh fruit and vegetables, and fresh fish, chicken and lean meat, should be substituted.

Practice Point – Incidence

- Hypertension is found in 70% of patients with NIDDM

Gestational diabetes

If diabetes mellitus is diagnosed for the first time during pregnancy then it is possible that the patient has longstanding non-insulin dependent diabetes mellitus. If the diabetes remits after the end of the pregnancy then the patient can be considered to have had gestational diabetes. However, half of all patients classified as having gestational diabetes will develop NIDDM within 15 years.[10] Many of these patients are obese or gain excessive amounts of weight during pregnancy and many are hypertensive. As with patients with IDDM, weight control without extreme dietary restriction and in some cases insulin therapy, are necessary. If the blood pressure is raised then the therapeutic choice is the same as in patients with IDDM.

Intrinsic Renal Disease

Renal diseases (principally glomerulonephritis and pyelonephritis) are the commonest causes of secondary hypertension in pregnancy. If renal function is severely impaired patients may be subfertile and generally unwell. Many women are found to have impaired renal function for the first time when they become pregnant and they need investigation with renal ultrasonography, creatinine clearance estimations, quantification of proteinuria, and a glucose tolerance test. Renal biopsy is occasionally necessary in pregnancy if renal function is very poor or deteriorating. There have been several reports of an irreversible deterioration of renal function during pregnancy, mainly in women with pre-existing renal impairment. Women with normal renal function but with evidence of glomerulonephritis may have a better outlook with no greater deterioration of renal function than comparable women who are not pregnant.[11] Women with IgA nephropathy, membranoproliferative glomerulonephritis, and those with focal segmental sclerosing glomerular lesions, may be at greater risk than those with membranous glomerulonephritis alone. Some patients with significant renal impairment due to glomerulonephritis may be treated with corticosteroids and immunosuppressive drugs including azathioprine. Furthermore, the ACE inhibitors are now increasingly being used in non-diabetic patients with nephropathy. Women of childbearing potential need to be advised of the hazards of these drugs in pregnancy. There are no convincing data on the effects of immunosuppressive drugs on fetal development, but they should be discontinued if at all possible. The management of these patients needs to be in close collaboration with a nephrologist.

In all renal syndromes in pregnancy, serum creatinine levels should be monitored at least monthly. There is a 50% chance the mother will develop pre-eclampsia, and intrauterine growth retardation is common, so regular obstetrical monitoring is necessary.[12] Patients with pyelonephritis and bilaterally scarred kidneys have a 50% chance of developing pre-eclampsia. They are not normally prescribed any specific medication although some nephrologists nowadays prescribe ACE inhibitors in order to preserve renal function. Many patients will be on continuous antibiotic therapy and regular urine microscopy and culture is necessary to detect new infections. Careful monitoring of renal function and fetal growth must be maintained.

Autosomal dominant polycystic kidney disease

This condition may remain undiagnosed until pregnancy. Pregnant women with a very strong family history of hypertension, renal failure, and both subarachnoid and intracerebral haemorrhage should be investigated by renal ultrasonography. If polycystic disease is diagnosed, patients should be advised that their children have a 50% chance of inheriting the disease. In view of the fact that polycystic disease can carry a good prognosis with appropriate treatment, termination of pregnancy is not justified.[13] In pregnancy, blood pressure control must be assiduous, maintaining pressures persistently below 140/90 mmHg, as the mother is at risk of subarachnoid haemorrhage, particularly during labour. Elective caesarean section should be seriously considered. In the autosomal dominant form of polycystic kidney disease the fetus does not have enlarged kidneys.

Practice Point – Renal Syndromes

- Patients with renal syndromes should have their serum creatinine levels monitored monthly
- There is a 50% chance that the mother will develop PET or IUGR

Adrenal Hypertension

Both primary hyperaldosteronism (Conn's syndrome) and phaeochromocytoma are often present in young people, and both conditions may not be diagnosed until pregnancy occurs. There is little information about Conn's syndrome in pregnancy. The diagnostic markers are unprovoked hypokalaemia with relatively raised serum sodium levels. Plasma aldosterone levels are usually very high and renin release is suppressed. The optimum method of managing this condition in pregnancy is unknown. It seems sensible to avoid spironolactone owing to its oestrogenic properties. Beta-blockers would be expected to be ineffective whereas thiazide diuretics may worsen hypokalaemia and even cause paralysis due to muscle weakness. The alpha-blockers and the dihydropyridine calcium channel blockers should be effective. Once the pregnancy is over the adrenal glands should be imaged by CT or MRI scanning to identify the small (1 cm) adrenal tumour which causes Conn's syndrome.

Phaeochromocytoma is well documented in pregnancy, with reports of both maternal and fetal death.[14] All women with significant hypertension in pregnancy should be screened for phaeochromocytoma even if they are symptomless, with one or more 24 hour urine collections for catecholamine excretion. Some drugs, including particularly methyldopa, may cause false positive results with urinary vanillylmandelic acid (VMA) but usually there is no interference with the metanephrines, adrenaline, noradrenaline or dopamine. If phaeochromocytoma is diagnosed, the tumour should be localised by abdominal ultrasound. Magnetic resonance imaging has been reported to be safe in pregnancy but should be reserved for patients where ultrasonography has been inconclusive. Antihypertensive treatment should be started urgently with the alpha-blocker phenoxybenzamine, if necessary in high doses to secure perfect blood pressure control and to reduce the intense vasoconstriction which characterises this condition. The beta-blocker propranolol, should only then be added in to control any tachycardia.[15] Delivery should be by elective caesarean section with a general surgeon and an expert anaesthetic team present. Some authorities recommend the removal of the tumour at the time of the caesarean section, whereas others would prefer a later operation through a more suitable abdominal incision. During operative procedures there may be violent swings in the blood pressure and pulse rate although these can be minimised with adequate preoperative alpha- and beta-blockade.

Connective Tissue Diseases

Both systemic lupus erythematosus (SLE) and polyarteritis nodosa are associated with renal damage and the development of hypertension. This problem is aggravated by the use of corticosteroids to modify the disease. SLE is also associated with fetal defects, including complete heart block due to failure of development of the His–Purkinje system.[16] When pregnancy occurs, ACE inhibitors and immunosuppressive drugs should be stopped and corticosteroid doses reduced with titration against laboratory indices of disease activity (C-reactive protein, plasma viscosity, urinary protein and serum creatinine).

The use of hydralazine on a long term basis is associated with the development of a lupus-like syndrome. In short term use in pregnancy it has not been reported to cause this problem.

Practice Point – Drugs

- The use of hydralazine in the long term is associated with a lupus-like syndrome in some patients

---

Aortic Coarctation

Coarctation of the aorta is usually diagnosed and corrected in childhood, particularly if there are associated congenital heart defects. However, some patients are not diagnosed until adult life and some present for the first time in pregnancy.[17] All women with hypertension in the first half of pregnancy should be checked for this condition by examining them for radiofemoral delay, and if there is any discrepancy, measurement of the blood pressure in the legs. This is done using a thigh cuff and with the stethoscope placed in the popliteal fossa. Beta-blocking drugs are considered to be the preferred option for controlling the blood pressure because they may reduce shear stress on the aortic wall which is prone to dissection or rupture. Surgical correction or balloon dilatation for coarctation is rarely necessary in pregnancy if the fetus can be demonstrated to be growing normally.

References

1 Mogensen CE, Christensen CK. Predicting diabetic nephropathy in insulin dependent patients. *N. Engl J Med* 1984;**311**:89–93.
2 Diabetes in pregnancy. *Clin Obstet Gynaecol* 1981;**24**:1–162.
3 Lewis EJ, Hunsicker LG *et al*. The effect of angiotensin-converting-enzyme inhibition on diabetic nephropathy. *N Engl J Med* 1993;**329**:1456–62.
4 Chaturevedi N, Sjolie A-K, Stephenson JH *et al* and the EUCLID Study Group. Effect of lisinopril in progression of retinopathy in normotensive people with type 1 diabetes. *Lancet* 1998;**351**:28–31.
5 Shotan A, Widerhorn J, Hurst A, Elkayan U. Risks of angiotensin converting enzyme inhibition in pregnancy; experimental and clinical evidence, potential mechanisms and recommendations for use. *Am J Med* 1994;**96**:451–6.
6 Lip GYH, Churchill D, Beevers M, Auckett A, Beevers DG. Angiotensin converting enzyme inhibitors in early pregnancy. *Lancet* 1997;**350**:1466–7.
7 Lip GYH, Beevers M, Churchill D, Shaffer LM, Beevers DG. Effect of atenolol on birth weight. *Am J Cardiol* 1997;**79**:1436–8.
8 Ferriss JB. The causes of raised blood pressure in insulin dependent and non-insulin dependent diabetes mellitus. *J Hum Hypertens* 1991;**5**:245–54.
9 Maxwell MH, Waks AU, Schroth PC, Karam M, Dornfield LP. Error in blood pressure measurement due to incorrect cuff size in obese patients. *Lancet* 1982;**2**:33–6.
10 Symposium on Gestational Diabetes. *Diabetes Care* 1980;**3**:399–501.
11 Jungers P, Houillier P, Forget D *et al*. Influence of pregnancy on the course of primary chronic glomerulonephritis. *Lancet* 1995;**346**:1122–4.
12 Surian M, Ibascia E *et al*. Glomerular disease in pregnancy: a study of 132 pregnancies in patients with primary and secondary glomerular disease. *Nephrology* 1984;**36**:101–5.
13 Gabow PA, Johnson AM, Kaeling WD *et al*. Factors affecting the progression of renal disease in autosomal dominant polycystic kidney disease. *Kid Int* 1992;**41**:1311–19.
14 Lamming GC, Symonds EM, Rubin PC. Phaeochromocytoma in pregnancy: still a cause of maternal death. *Clin Exp Hypertens* 1990;**9**:57–68.
15 Harper MA, Murnaghan GA, Kennedy L *et al* Phaeochromocytoma in pregnancy. Five cases and a review of literature. *Br J Obstet Gynaecol* 1989;**96**:594–606.
16 Hughes GRV, Gharavi AE. The anticardiolipin syndrome. *J Rheumatol* 1986;**13**:486–9.
17 Deal K, Wolley CF. Coarctation of the aorta and pregnancy. *Ann Intern Med* 1973;**78**:706–10.

9 Postpartum Follow-up of Hypertension in Pregnancy

DG BEEVERS AND D CHURCHILL

All women who have had any form of hypertension in pregnancy should be followed up carefully, although in most patients, only one postnatal visit is necessary. Women who have had pre-eclampsia and who have required antihypertensive drugs should have these withdrawn gradually. Occasionally in the postpartum phase some women may sustain a sharp rise in blood pressure and an increase in proteinuria. This is an uncommon event, mimicking pre-eclampsia, which is not to be expected because delivery of the placenta usually results in rapid normalisation of blood pressure, but there are occasional exceptions.

Once pregnancy is over most women should be reviewed by a clinician after about 6 weeks. Those who suffered from pre-eclampsia will almost always have normalised their blood pressures at this stage. No action is necessary other than counselling the patient on the risks of hypertension in future pregnancies. Many will not develop pre-eclampsia in later pregnancies. Although there is uncertainty whether pre-eclampsia is related to hypertension in later life, it seems prudent to advise regular blood pressure checks as the years go by, and particularly at the time of the menopause.[1]

All women affected by pre-eclampsia, together with those with no known chronic hypertension but whose blood pressures have not settled should be checked to exclude any underlying cause for their hypertension. Urinary catecholamines, if not already tested, should be measured in a 24 hour urine collection. At this stage abdominal ultrasonography to examine renal size and shape may be a little misleading. Dilatation of the ureters and renal pelvis may occur as the result of a gravid uterus in the lower abdomen, thus giving the erroneous impression of hydronephrosis. Renal imaging should therefore be postponed until about 8 weeks postpartum.

It is also important to follow up women with known chronic or pre-existing hypertension 6 weeks postpartum. Long term anti-hypertensive drug therapy in low risk pre-menopausal women is definitely necessary if the blood pressure consistently exceeds 160/100 mmHg. In women with diastolic pressures between 90 and 99 mmHg, careful observation with regular reinforcement of non-pharmacological advice on controlling hypertension is necessary. In particular, weight gain in pregnancy should be reversed and salt restriction instituted.

There are very few women who should be advised not to become pregnant again on medical grounds. The main group are those with intrinsic renal disease who have impaired renal function (serum creatinine of 180 μmol/l or more). In these, the hazards of pregnancy should be explained. Some may opt to have further children on the grounds that they know they are going to develop end stage renal failure within a few years anyway, so the risks of hastening this event are offset by the wish to have a family. The patient's view is paramount as long as it is based on information provided in a sensitive manner by a sympathetic clinician.

The issue of contraception also needs addressing in the postpartum period. There is probably a small extra risk that women who have had pre-eclampsia or "gestational" hypertension will develop raised blood pressure whilst taking oral contraceptives. The risk may be greater in women with chronic or pre-existing hypertension.[2] However, with careful monitoring, the use of low oestrogen or progesterone only compounds, taken together with the avoidance of weight gain and cigarette smoking, the risk is small – much less than the hazards of an unwanted pregnancy in a high-risk woman.

Children of Mothers with Hypertensive Pregnancy

Women who have had severe hypertension in pregnancy or who developed pre-eclampsia tend to give birth to small babies. Often they are born well before term, sometimes after induction of labour or caesarean section. Their immediate risk in the neonatal period is respiratory distress syndrome. However, there is now evidence that these babies are more prone to develop hypertension themselves in later life and it has thus been postulated that intrauterine under-nutrition may play an important role in cardiovascular disease.[3] It is unlikely that the hypothesis explains the inverse relationship observed between maternal blood pressure and fetal weight which is seen in entirely healthy mothers and babies in the 1990s. It is possible that women with a tendency towards essential hypertension do tend to give birth to smaller babies, who inherit the tendency to develop hypertension in later life. Thus, the concordance of blood pressure in families is both environmental as well as genetic.[4] From a practical point of view the clinician merely needs to be aware that hypertension runs in families.

Practice Point – Follow-up

- All women who suffer hypertension during pregnancy should have careful follow-up 6 weeks after delivery
- Treatment should be withdrawn gradually
- If the blood pressure is not normal 6 weeks post delivery, the patient should be investigated to exclude an underlying cause for her hypertension
- Non-pharmacological advice is as important as drug therapy

References

1 Fisher KA, Luger A, Spargo BH, Lindheimer MD. Hypertension in pregnancy: clinico-pathological correlations and remote prognosis. *Medicine* 1981;**60**:267–72.

2 Fisch IR, Freedman SH, Myatt AV. Oral contraceptives, pregnancy and blood pressure. *J Am Med Assoc* 1972;**22**:1507–10.

3 Barker DJP, Osmond C, Golding J, Kuh D, Wadsworth WEJ. Growth in utero, blood pressure in childhood and adult life and mortality from cardiovascular disease. *Br Med J* 1989;**289**:564–7.

4 Churchill D, Perry IJ, Beevers DG. Ambulatory blood pressure in pregnancy and fetal growth. *Lancet* 1997:**349**:7–10.

Appendix:
Patient Support Groups

Action on Pre-eclampsia (APEC)
31–33 College Road
Harrow
Middlesex
HA1 1EJ

Telephone 0181 863 3271 Fax 0181 424 0653 Helpline 01923
266778

British Hypertension Society Information Service
Blood Pressure Unit
St George's Hospital Medical School
Cranmer Terrace
London
SW17 0RE

Telephone 0181 725 3412 Fax 0181 725 2959

Miscarriage Association
c/o Clayton Hospital
Northgate
Wakefield
West Yorkshire
WF1 3JS

Telephone 01924 200799

Stillbirth & Neonatal Death Society (SANDS)
28 Portland Place
London
W1N 4NE

Telephone 0171 436 5881/7940 Fax 0171 436 3715

Support Around Termination for Abnormality (SATFA)
73–75 Charlotte Street
London
W1P 1LB

Telephone 0171 631 0285

Index

Note: Pages numbers in **bold** refer to figures, those in *italic* refer to tables or boxed material.

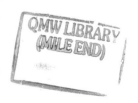